Pharmacoepidemiology and Pharmacovigilance

Pharmacoepidemiology and Pharmacovigilance

Synergistic Tools to Better Investigate Drug Safety

Sabrina Nour

Gilles Plourde

ACADEMIC PRESS
An imprint of Elsevier

Academic Press is an imprint of Elsevier
125 London Wall, London EC2Y 5AS, United Kingdom
525 B Street, Suite 1650, San Diego, CA 92101, United States
50 Hampshire Street, 5th Floor, Cambridge, MA 02139, United States
The Boulevard, Langford Lane, Kidlington, Oxford OX5 1GB, United Kingdom

Notices
Knowledge and best practice in this field are constantly changing. As new research and experience broaden our understanding, changes in research methods, professional practices, or medical treatment may become necessary.

Practitioners and researchers must always rely on their own experience and knowledge in evaluating and using any information, methods, compounds, or experiments described herein. In using such information or methods they should be mindful of their own safety and the safety of others, including parties for whom they have a professional responsibility.

To the fullest extent of the law, neither the Publisher nor the authors, contributors, or editors, assume any liability for any injury and/or damage to persons or property as a matter of products liability, negligence or otherwise, or from any use or operation of any methods, products, instructions, or ideas contained in the material herein.

Library of Congress Cataloging-in-Publication Data
A catalog record for this book is available from the Library of Congress

British Library Cataloguing-in-Publication Data
A catalogue record for this book is available from the British Library

ISBN: 978-0-12-816183-8

Publisher: Mica H. Haley
Acquisition Editor: Kattie Washington
Editorial Project Manager: Sam W. Young
Production Project Manager: Mohanapriyan Rajendran
Designer: Mark Rogers

Typeset by TNQ Technologies

Contents

Biography

Sabrina Nour is a clinical evaluator for BGTD at Health Canada. In this role she is in charge of reviewing the efficacy and safety of biological products. She also holds a Master of Science degree in Epidemiology and a certification in Population Health and Risk Assessment Management, both from the University of Ottawa. She is particularly interested in Pharmacoepidemiology, pharmacovigilance, and the influence of health policies on populations.

Dr. Plourde is a senior clinical evaluator of biological products for the Biologic and Genetic Therapies Directorate (BGTD) at Health Canada (Canada's food and drug regulatory agency). He is an associate professor with the Department of Clinical Pharmacology and Physiology at the University of Montreal and with the School of Physical Activity Sciences at the University of Ottawa's Faculty of Medicine. He holds a doctorate in medicine from the University of Montreal and a Ph.D. in experimental medicine from Laval University, dealing with the physiology involved in type 1 diabetes drug development. His studies led him to publish several articles in highly rated scientific journals, and he has made numerous presentations for prestigious associations at National and International levels. Dr. Plourde has also supervised many students and employees interested in the management of adverse drug reactions of biological products both in clinical research and/or when health products have obtained marketing authorization.

Foreword

Drugs have certainly changed the way we approach, treat, and manage a variety of health problems. Despite their benefits, they can also cause different health problems, disabilities, extended hospital stays, or even death; however, it is imperative to notice that the adverse reactions they cause are often preventable.[1,2]

In several countries, adverse drug reactions are among the top 10 leading causes of mortality, illustrating the importance of dealing with the prevention of this safety issue as efficiently as possible. For example, adverse drug reactions are classified between the fourth and the sixth leading cause of mortality in the United States. Based on an average fatality of 106,000 deaths, it was found that drug-related mortality was ranked fourth, just behind heart disease (743,460 deaths), cancer (529,904 deaths), and stroke (150,108 deaths) and before pulmonary disease (101,077 deaths).[3] Ross Baker et al.[4] suggested that 7.5% of patients admitted to hospitals for acute care in Canada for the fiscal year 2000 experienced one or more adverse drug reactions, and among them 36.9% were potentially preventable.

A metaanalysis conducted in 2002 has also shown that 4.9% of hospital admissions were associated with adverse drug reactions, although estimates vary anywhere from 0.2% to 41.3% based on individual studies.[5] According to this metaanalysis, 28.9% of the adverse drug reactions leading to hospitalizations were considered preventable.

In 2012, another metaanalysis,[6] which excluded adverse drug reactions associated with nonadherence and overdose, consisting of 16 studies among 48,797 patients presenting to the emergency department or admitted to hospital and 8 studies involving 24,128 patients already admitted in the hospital demonstrated that 2% (95% confidence interval [CI]: 1.2%−3.2%) of patients presenting to the emergency department or admitted to hospital had adverse drug reactions, and 52% (95% CI: 42%−62%) of these adverse drug reactions could have been avoided.

Among the 8 studies involving patients already admitted in the hospital, 1.6% (95% CI: 0.1%−51%) had adverse drug reactions, including 45% (95% CI: 33%−58%) that could have, once again, been avoided. This metaanalysis demonstrated that adverse drug reactions are a significant cause of morbidity in patients, whether or not they are admitted to the hospital and about 50% of these patients had adverse drugs reactions that could have been avoided.

Thomsen et al.[7] have shown, using a systematic review of 29 studies, that adverse drug reactions are also common in ambulatory patients and that many of these adverse drug reactions may result in hospitalizations that could have been avoided.

This study is in agreement with the results of a previous study, carried out by Pirmohamed M. et al.,[8] which showed a high risk of adverse drug reactions also in ambulatory patients and suggests that measures must be taken to prevent these adverse drug reactions at different levels of the health-care system (including patients seen at the emergency department because nearly one out of every nine visits to the emergency room are due to an adverse drug reaction, and up to 68% of these incidents are considered avoidable).

In short, the preventability of adverse drug reactions in hospitalized patients or patients seen at the emergency or in an ambulatory setting justifies the need to put in place measures to better prevent adverse drug reactions throughout a product's entire life cycle. Our aim in this book is to discuss how principles of pharmacoepidemiology combined with pharmacovigilance may be particularly helpful in the analysis and management of these adverse drug reactions.

Recent studies have shown that adverse drug reactions are responsible for a third of the cases of hospitalization with an average length of stay in the hospital of 3.1 days.[9,10] The proportion of hospitalizations from adverse drug reactions can reach, in some countries, from 10% to 20% of the health budget that is allocated to expenses related to complications caused by drugs.[8,11,12]

The cost of morbidity and mortality related to drugs in the United States amounted to more than 177.4 billion USD for the year 2001. Since 1995, the costs associated with problems related to adverse drug reactions have more than doubled; in fact the costs related to the morbidity and mortality associated with drugs exceed the cost of the drugs themselves.[13]

The latest estimates from the World Health Organization (WHO) reveal similar impacts related to adverse drug reactions in other countries that spend also between 15% and 20% of their health budget on problems related to drugs, suggesting that this phenomenon is not only present in the Canada or the United States but is also prevalent worldwide.

Without neglecting the impact of some scandals and tragedies (Thalidomide 1962, Meridia 2010, Vioxx 2004, and Raptiva 2009) on public opinion and on consumer confidence in our health-care systems.[14] The main objective of this book is to discuss strategies for the prevention of the adverse effects of the health product throughout the life cycle of these products to provide various partners—universities, doctors, pharmacists, nurses, and the public in general—with the tools that may enable safer use of health products. The goal is also to enable patients to make informed decisions related to the use of these products, as well as to increase the public's confidence in our health-care system.

The majority of impacts induced by adverse drug reactions can be significantly reduced through the application of integrated strategies of drug safety surveillance using an ongoing assessment of the risk/benefit ratio according to the life cycle of the product. This can be achieved in the context of greater activity in the prevention of adverse drug reactions and by making better use of the pharmacoepidemiology and pharmacovigilance tools we already have.

The birth of pharmacoepidemiology and pharmacovigilance can be dated back to the early 1960s. Growing concerns regarding adverse drug reactions emphasized the need to develop methods to study the safety of drug therapy, not only in premarketing but also in postmarketing settings.

Obviously, the **thalidomide** disaster in the late 1950s and others in the early 1960s strengthened the requirements for the pharmaceutical industry to provide proof of the safety of their health products before and after approval. In 1960, the Federal Drug Administration (FDA), the European Medical Agency (EMA), Health Canada, WHO, and other regulatory agencies started collecting adverse drug reaction reports. These systems were further developed, and the terms pharmacoepidemiology and pharmacovigilance were proposed as new disciplines.

During the last decades of the 20th century, pharmacoepidemiology and pharmacovigilance shifted from being focused entirely on adverse drug reactions found in both pre- and postmarket settings and risk association studies, to also include other clinical outcomes and health economic aspects of drug use.

To prepare this book, we first conducted a literature search, which mainly covered relevant literature published between January 2006 and January 2017. Our research focused on the following topics: (1) prevention of the side effects of health products, (2) pharmacovigilance and pharmacoepidemiology, and (3) the life cycle of health products, biologics, pharmaceuticals, biosimilars, and generic products. We selected the most recent articles to better reflect current knowledge.

Selected documents come from a consultation with Scopus, Medline, and in certain situations in consultation with the database of Cochrane systematic reviews. This book is supplemented by a brief discussion of the various guidance documents from Health Canada, FDA, EMA, WHO, the International Conference on Harmonisation (ICH), and other organizations.

In the context of this book, we do not have the goal of presenting the content of all of these guidance documents but rather to bring out the essence of these documents so that the readers can use them as reference tools, to improve their knowledge and understanding of the topics discussed in this book. These various guidance documents are presented at the end of the book, allowing readers to have electronic access should they wish to further supplement their understanding with additional detail.

REFERENCES

1. Brennan TA, Leape LL, Laird MM, et al. Incidence of adverse events and negligence in hospitalized patients. Results of the Harvard Medical Practice Study 1. *N Eng J Med.* 1991;324:370–377.
2. Wilson RM, Runciman WB, Gibberd RW, et al. The quality in Australian Health Care Study. *Med J Aust.* 1995;163:458–476.
3. Lazarou J, Pomeranz BH, Corey PN. Incidence of adverse drug reactions in hospitalized patients: a meta-analysis of prospective studies. *J Am Med Assoc.* 1998;279:1200–1205.
4. Ross Baker G, Norton PG, Flintoft V, et al. The Canadian Adverse Event Study: the incidence of adverse events among hospital patients in Canada. *CMAJ.* 2004;170:1668–1686.
5. Beijer HJ, de Blacy CJ. Hospitalisation caused by adverse drug reactions (ADR): a meta-analysis of observational studies. *Pharm World Sci.* 2002;24:46–54.
6. Hakkarainen KM, Hedna K, Petzold M, Hagg S. Percentage of patients with preventable adverse drug reactions and preventability of adverse drug reactions: a meta-analysis. *PLoS One.* 2012:1–9.
7. Thomssen LA, Winterstein AG, Sondergaard B, et al. Systematic review of the incidence and characteristics of preventable adverse drug events in ambulatory care. *Ann Phramacother.* 2007;41:1411–1426.
8. Pirmohamed M, James S, Meakin S, et al. Adverse drug reactions as cause of admission to hospital: prospective analysis of 18 820 patients. *BMJ.* 2004;329:15–19.
9. Classen DC, Resar R, Griffin F, et al. 'Global Trigger Tool' shows that adverse events in hospitals may be ten times greater than previously measured. *Health Aff.* 2011;30:581–589.
10. Hug BL, Keohane C, Seger DL, et al. The cost of adverse drug events in community hospital. *J Comm J Qual Patient Saf.* 2012;38:120–126.
11. Patel H, et al. Trends in hospital admissions for adverse drug reactions in England: analysis of national hospital episode statistics 1998–2005. *BMC Clinical Pharmacology.* 2007;7:9.
12. Imbs J, Pouyanne P, Haramburu F, et al. Adverse drug reactions : prevalence in French public hospitals. *Therapie.* 1999;52:21–27.
13. Ernst FR, Grizzle AJ. Drug-related morbidity and mortality: updating the cost-of-ilness model. *J Am Pharm Assoc.* 2001;41:192–199.
14. Herder M, Gibson E, Graham J, et al. Regulating prescription drugs for patient safety: does Bill C-17 go far enough? *CMAJ.* 2014;186:E287–E292.

Chapter 1

Introduction

Epidemiology refers to a scientific discipline that uses knowledge from the biological sciences, social sciences, the theory of probabilities, and statistical tools to study and quantify the presence and causes of health problems in humans.[1–4] Although various definitions have been proposed to describe the word "epidemiology," the common theme that emerges from almost all of these definitions is that the study of epidemiologic data serves three main objectives:

(1) Epidemiology is often used *for descriptive purposes* to describe the distribution and frequency of a health problem in humans or among specific subgroups of the population.
(2) It is also commonly used *for analytic purposes* to identify the causes and risk factors of many health problems.
(3) It is also used *for assessment purposes* to assess the results of an intervention on a specific health problem in a specific subpopulation.[2,5–6]

For a thorough introduction to the concepts of epidemiology, the reader is invited to consult the following books: *Modern Epidemiology (3rd ed.)* by Rothman et al. and *Epidemiology for the Uninitiated (5th ed.)* by Coggon et al.[1]

Notice that the definition of epidemiology is purposefully kept broad since it has a large scope with major applications for the study of a variety of health issues, thus creating smaller but more focused branches. For instance, pharmacoepidemiology is one such branch and will be the focus of this book. A comprehensive definition of pharmacoepidemiology is found in the fifth edition of the book *A Dictionary of Epidemiology*, and it is defined as: "*The study of the distribution and determinants of drug-related events in populations and the application of this study to efficacious treatment. The application of epidemiological knowledge, methods, and reasoning is to describe, explain, control and predict the uses and effects (beneficial and adverse) of drugs, vaccines and related biological products in human populations [...]. P"harmacoepidemiology also aids pharmacology, public health, and other health sciences by increasing knowledge about the occurrence and causes of diseases, the distribution of health states and the functioning of the healthcare system.*"[2]

Pharmacoepidemiology and Pharmacovigilance. https://doi.org/10.1016/B978-0-12-816183-8.00001-9

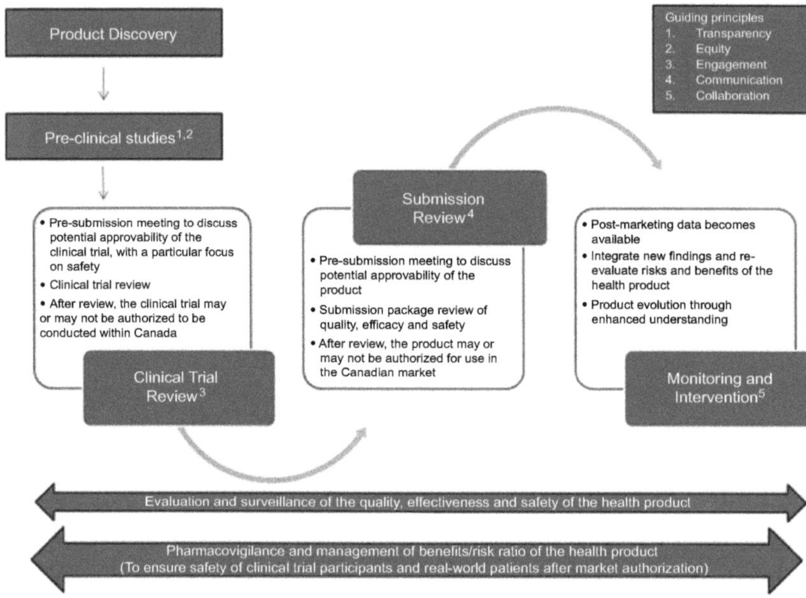

FIGURE 1.1 Product life cycle. 1, The OCDE Good Laboratory Practices (GLP): The OCDE GLP is the study of the molecule, its effect on cells of animals, target organs and other aspects related to the management of preclinical studies including data analyzing, archiving, planning, publication, and other aspects related to laboratory activities. This first point also includes GLP inspection to ensure quality, reproducibility, and the integrity of the results regarding the efficacy and safety of chemical or biological substances. It also includes best practices from Health Canada's Good Manufacturing Practice (GMP) and GMP inspection to ensure the quality of the material chosen for the production and to ensure that the techniques of packaging, labeling, analysis, distribution, import, and sales meet the established standards. (For more information the reader is invited to consult these Guidelines at the Resources for Readers section). 2, Additional tools: these tools are the ICH M3 (R2) and S6 (R1) Guidelines on preclinical safety evaluation for pharmaceutical and biotechnology products, respectively. There are various other ICH guidelines discussing preclinical safety studies (pharmacology, target organ toxicity, reproductive toxicity, genotoxicity, carcinogenicity, maximum tolerated dose, without toxic effects, and others) http://www.ich.org/products/guidelines/safety/article/safety-guidelines.html (this information is used to estimate an initial safe dose for clinical trials in humans and to identify parameters for medical follow-up of potential adverse effects). 3, Good Clinical Practice of Division 5 of the Food and Drug Regulations, the ICH E6 on Good Clinical Practice Guidelines and Inspection Guidelines: These measures are meant to ensure and verify the validity of the data presented on the clinical, pharmacological, pharmacokinetic, or pharmacodynamic effects of drugs for human use to detect and require the report of adverse reactions and to study the absorption, distribution, metabolism, efficacy, and efficiency. This also contains the recommendations of the ICH E2A Guidelines on the mandatory reporting to Health Canada of all serious and unexplained adverse reactions observed in clinical trials. The goal is to ensure the safety of clinical trials participants. 4, Division 8 of the Food and Drug Regulations and the Management of Health Canada Drug Submission Guidelines: These tools are used to determine what must be submitted and evaluated to confirm the quality, efficacy, and safety (favorable benefit/risk ratio) of a health product for marketing authorization purposes and includes (1) basic scientific information about the health product; (2) the aspects related to the quality of the product; (3) preclinical studies; (4) clinical efficacy and safety of a

As mentioned, pharmacoepidemiology includes the study of the use and effects of health products in populations. As it will be discussed in this book, the designs used in pharmacoepidemiologic studies are not much different from those used in other areas of clinical epidemiology. However, there are three key differences between both statistical sciences and this will be discussed below:

(1) Because pharmacoepidemiologic studies are usually performed after a health product has been approved for marketing, and because around 500–3000 patients are generally studied during the premarket phase (before approval), pharmacoepidemiologic studies usually must include substantially larger numbers of patients (depending on the indication) that must be followed for a longer duration to add new useful information;

(2) Because at least one randomized control trial (RCT) (or a pivotal trial) was already performed prior to drug marketing, pharmacoepidemiologic studies are less likely to use RCT study designs because many of the same limitations, which the premarketing RCTs were subject to, would apply as well as to any postmarketing RCT and therefore would not contribute adding new useful information. For example, because RCTs are not an efficient means of studying uncommon adverse effects, the drug effects in patients are commonly excluded from such trials;

(3) Because, pharmacoepidemiologic questions often arise from regulatory and public health concerns, answers must often be obtained very quickly. This need for rapidly performed studies of massive sample size has led to a series of special approaches that have characterized the field of pharmacoepidemiology.

The second partner involved in the management of adverse drug reactions is pharmacovigilance. This component is defined as being the science and

health product; (5) an analysis of the benefit/risk ratio; (6) a product monograph labeling and patient's information leaflet; (7) a risk management plan, including the pharmacovigilance plan, if necessary. After approval the manufacturer must take the necessary measures to ensure that the benefit/risk ratio remains favorable and the risks can be mitigated, managed, and warned throughout the product life cycle by a passive and active surveillance of the adverse drug reactions, by the reporting of safety report synthesis annually or on request (risk management plan, periodic benefit–risk evaluation report, and development safety update report) and by providing additional studies on specific populations including post–market phase IV studies, registries, and others (discussed below). 5, Good pharmacovigilance practice and Inspections: These tools are used to monitor the safety, efficacy, and quality of drugs after the marketing approval. This activity consists in monitoring, prevention, and reassessment of adverse drug reactions and must conform to the Food and Drug Regulations (see sections C.01.016 to C.01.020) that require the manufacturers to report adverse reactions to Health Canada and any product failure in a timely manner according to their severity and novelty as well as all changes in the benefit/risk ratio of a health product. As a result of this monitoring activity terms of use can be changed and modified, suspended, or even authorization revoked by the Minister. The goal is to ensure the safety of patients during real-world use.

activities relating to the detection, assessment, understanding, and prevention of adverse effects or any other safety problem related to health products on the market (intolerance to drugs, unauthorized use or misuse, therapeutic error, drug dependence, drug resistance, drug abuse, and others). Please consult the glossary of pharmacovigilance terms at the end of Chapter 2 to have a more in-depth understanding of terms related to pharmacovigilance.

To reduce adverse drug reactions, regulatory authorities such as Health Canada, FDA, EMA, and others regulatory authorities have developed pharmacovigilance programs for the evaluation, control, and monitoring of these adverse drug reactions, including the monitoring programs in postapproval phase. Again, the information included in the glossary at the end of Annex 1 would be relevant to consolidate the information discussed about pharmacovigilance.

It is well known that many adverse drug reactions remain unknown for years following marketing of a health product. Therefore, it is essential to learn more about their use in the long term and in specific population groups. Usually, people who are at high risk because of their age (such as young children and the elderly), a special situation (pregnant or breast-feeding women or persons of different racial or ethnic origin), a particular condition (the carriers of genetic polymorphisms), or their health status (complex pathology, polypharmacy) are generally excluded from clinical trial protocols. However, all these patients may receive the drug when it becomes available on the market, hence the importance of setting up an effective pharmacovigilance program for them. It is therefore essential that new health products are subject to a control of efficacy and safety in real conditions of use, i.e., after their authorization for marketing and throughout their life cycle using an adequate pharmacovigilance program (see Fig. 1.1).

This book provides a summary review of the various epidemiologic tools or study designs commonly used for the passive and active surveillance of drug-related adverse effects, including a discussion of the strengths and weaknesses of each tool and design.

The main criticisms surrounding pharmacoepidemiologic research will also be examined and we will focus on issues related to bias and confounding factors that often interfere in conducting these studies as well as in the interpretation of the data obtained from these studies.

We will also provide a brief description on the databases used in pharmacoepidemiologic research including a discussion on their strengths and weaknesses. It is important to note that the information related to pharmacoepidemiology and pharmacovigilance discussed in this book will be consolidated by providing short glossaries of terms of both activities at the end of their respective chapters.

We will finish this book by providing case reports to further illustrate, in a more concrete way, the synergistic role of pharmacoepidemiology and pharmacovigilance in the management of adverse drug reactions. Each case report illustrates a real situation (no confidential data are reported) and is composed of questions and answers based on appropriate clinical situations to provide all the necessary tools to better manage adverse drug reactions.

REFERENCES

1. Coggon D, Rose G, Barker D. *Epidemiology for the Uninitiated.* 5th ed. London: BMJ; 2003.
2. Porta M, ed. *A Dictionary of Epidemiology.* 5th ed. New York: Oxford University Press; 2008.
3. Rothman KJ, Greenland S, Lash TL. In: Rothman KJ, ed. *Modern Epidemiology.* 3rd ed. Philadelphia, PA: Lippincott, Williams & Wilkins; 2008.
4. World Health Organization. http://www.who.int/topics/epidemiology/en/.
5. Strom B, Kimmel S, Hennessy Sean, eds. *Textbook of Pharmacoepidemiology.* 2nd ed. Sussex: John Wiley & Sons; 2013.
6. Yang Y, West-Strum D. *Understanding Pharmacoepidemiology.* New York: McGraw-Hill Medical; 2010.

Chapter 2

Pharmacovigilance

2.1 INTRODUCTION

Pharmacovigilance refers to the science and activities relating to the detection, assessment, understanding, and prevention of adverse effects and other drug-related safety problems. Related to this general definition, the underlying objectives of pharmacovigilance are to prevent harm from adverse reactions in humans that arise from the use of health products within or outside the terms of marketing authorization and in relation to the life cycle of these health products.

The main goal of pharmacovigilance is thus to promote the safe and effective use of health products, in particular by providing timely information about the safety of health products to patients, health-care professionals, and the public. Pharmacovigilance is therefore an activity contributing to the protection of patients and maintaining public health.

Many other issues are also of relevance to pharmacovigilance-related activities and include medication errors, lack of efficacy reports, off-label use, acute and chronic poisoning, assessment of drug-related mortality, abuse and misuse of health products, and adverse interactions of medicines with chemicals and other drugs (see Annex 1).

The pharmacovigilance approach can be clinical, epidemiological, experimental (e.g., to reproduce an adverse effect in animals to better understand the mechanism involved for human protection), or diagnostic (e.g., imputable methods).

The ultimate goal of pharmacovigilance is to accurately characterize and optimize the benefit/risk ratio of a health product throughout its life cycle.

2.2 OBJECTIVES OF PHARMACOVIGILANCE

Once available on the market, a drug leaves the scientific and restrictive environment of clinical trials and becomes legally available for consumption by the general public.

At the stage of clinical trials, however, most of the drugs have been assessed for both efficacy and safety for only a relatively short period of time and only on a relatively limited number of carefully selected patients (see also

Pharmacoepidemiology and Pharmacovigilance. https://doi.org/10.1016/B978-0-12-816183-8.00002-0

the short glossary in Annex 2 Annex that discusses the phases of development of a new drug and the selection of participants for each of these phases).

After being exposed to the monitoring recommended in clinical trials, it is therefore essential that new drugs are subject to a control of efficacy and safety in real conditions of use, i.e., after their authorization for marketing. Historical tragedies such as those mentioned earlier in the introductory chapter of this book remind us of the importance of these pharmacovigilance activities.

According to the World Health Organization (WHO) (2004), Eurasanté (2006), the Framework of Vigilance of Health Products (2012), and Dugair (2009), the main objectives of pharmacovigilance programs are (1) to improve the care and safety of patients and the general public; (2) to contribute to the assessment of the effectiveness and risks presented by health products and to encourage a safe, rational, and more effective use of these products (including on the economic point of view); and (3) to promote better education and training in this field to improve the effectiveness of communication between health-care professionals, patients, and the general public.[1–4]

2.3 PRODUCT LIFE CYCLE

According to what is presented in Fig. 1.1 of Chapter 1, a product's life cycle refers to a set of regulatory, administrative, and monitoring activities, which, at first view, may appear cumbersome and bureaucratic, but the concept is of major importance in the prevention of adverse drug reactions and in the maintenance of a positive benefit/risk ratio of a health product during its entire life.

Because this life cycle refers to all stages preceding and following the marketing of a health product, it includes the following steps:

- **(i)** the discovery of the product;
- **(ii)** the preclinical studies;
- **(iii)** the clinical trials;
- **(iv)** the presentation of product information by the manufacturer to the regulatory agency for its evaluation and approval;
- **(v)** the decision whether to allow the sale of the product;
- **(vi)** the distribution and sale of the product;
- **(vii)** the monitoring, inspection, and postmarketing investigations.

The ultimate goal is to ensure that patients have access to efficient and safe health products not only as participants during clinical trials but also in real life following the marketing authorization of these health products (see Fig. 1.1 of Chapter 1).[5,6] Fig. 1.1 of Chapter 1 shows the regulatory agencies monitoring activities as a variety of regulatory activities divided into a continuum. Thus, these activities can integrate and use information that continues to develop throughout the life cycle of a health product. The most relevant regulations surrounding the product life cycle are presented in one of the appendices at the end of this book.

To have a concrete picture of the product life cycle please also consult the case reports presented in Chapter 4.

2.4 PREVENTION TOOLS FOR PASSIVE AND ACTIVE SURVEILLANCE

The purpose of this section is to give a brief overview of some of the main pharmacovigilance tools for passive and active surveillance of adverse effects associated with drugs (see Chapter 4 for concrete examples on active and passive surveillance of adverse drug reactions).

Passive surveillance (pharmacovigilance) is mainly composed of spontaneous reports of adverse drug reactions, case series, and annual safety reports, whereas active surveillance (pharmacovigilance) is mainly composed of patient registries and pharmacoepidemiologic studies (pharmacoepidemiologic studies will be explained in greater detail in Chapter 3). Of note, we should not neglect passive surveillance as it is an excellent way to generate hypotheses for pharmacoepidemiologic studies.

2.5 PASSIVE SURVEILLANCE (PHARMACOVIGILANCE)

2.5.1 Spontaneous Reporting of Adverse Drug Reactions

A spontaneous report is an unsolicited communication from health-care professionals or consumers to a manufacturer, or a regulatory authority such as Health Canada, or other organizations such as the WHO, the Food and Drug Administration (FDA), the European Medical Agency (EMA), the regional centers, the poison centers, and others that describe one or more adverse reactions in a patient who was given one or more health products but is not part of a clinical study or any organized data collection system.

These spontaneous reports play a major role in the identification of postmarketing safety signals.[7] In many cases, a manufacturer or a regulatory agency can be alerted of rare adverse drug effects that were not detected during clinical trials or other studies in preauthorization phase. They may also contain important information on risk groups, risk factors, and the clinical characteristics of known serious adverse reactions. See Chapter 4 for other information on the role and use of spontaneous reporting (pharmacovigilance) in the identification of new safety signals. For more information on those terms, please also consult the glossary of pharmacovigilance terms in Annex 1.

According to Wise et al.,[8] reports of adverse reactions that occur when a health product is used in clinical practice form the basis of most drug-prevention systems and regulators use these databases to store and analyze reports of adverse events with the purpose of eventually doing a causality assessment of specific adverse drug reactions. For a definition of causality assessment, please consult the glossary of terms in Annex 2.

For example, the Medicines and Healthcare Products Regulatory Agency (MHRA) in United Kingdom operates a system of yellow cards for health-care professionals and patients to report adverse drug reactions and these reports are collected in the database of the MHRA.

The FDA runs a similar system in which reports of adverse events associated with drugs are stored in the AERS or the VAERS databases for reports of adverse events associated with vaccines.

Health Canada runs the Canada Vigilance database in which reports of adverse events associated with health products are stored. For your information, these systems are essentially considered passive systems. For more information and concrete examples on the usefulness of these databases, please see Chapter 4.

In other words, patients are not selected to participate in a specific database and reports are not actively solicited. These systems have the benefits of being able to be used throughout the health product life cycle.

They can be used to generate safety signals or to identify rare adverse effects associated with health products. Unfortunately, these databases cannot eliminate the risk of selection bias, correct low rates of reports, or reduce the high number of incomplete reports, thus limiting its ability to establish a causal relationship between a health product and an adverse effect.[8,9] This will be further discussed below.

That being said, we should certainly not neglect their potential in generating hypotheses of an association between exposure to a health product and a specific adverse effect that can then be confirmed with pharmacoepidemiologic studies. In short, these spontaneous case reports are the starting point of the adverse drug reaction pharmacovigilance activities: they are often the initial signal in prompting pharmacoepidemiologic studies.

To add efficiency in the spontaneous reporting of adverse drug reactions, it is essential to have the manufacturers, patients, and health-care professional collaboration in writing and sending detailed and good-quality reports to regulatory authorities including Health Canada (see below).

2.5.1.1 Identification of Safety Signals From Spontaneous Reporting

To compensate, at least up to a certain point, for the weaknesses inherent in the spontaneous reporting of adverse drug reactions, different epidemiologic techniques can be used for the identification of safety signals (see Chapter 3). These methods include the calculation of the disproportionality ratio, the use of Bayesian data exploration (data mining), and other techniques. However, these latest techniques should always be used in conjunction with the analysis of the individual case reports (for more concrete examples on the use of these pharmacoepidemiologic methods please consult the relevant case reports provided in Chapter 4).

Data-mining techniques facilitate the evaluation of spontaneous reports using statistical methods to detect potential signals to conduct a more in-depth safety assessment. These tools do not quantify the magnitude of the risk, and one must be careful when comparing health products.

The results obtained with these techniques should be interpreted considering also the weaknesses of the spontaneous reporting system and specifically, the major differences between the different health products. One should also consider the many biases and potential confounding factors that can also be associated to the spontaneous reporting of an adverse drug reaction.

All signals must be evaluated recognizing the possibility of false positives. In addition, the absence of a signal does not necessarily mean that there is no problem that needs to be followed.

2.5.2 Case Series Reports

Case series reports may also provide evidence of a link between a drug and an adverse effect, but they are also generally more useful to generate hypotheses of an association between exposure to a health product and an adverse effect, which can then be verified using one of the pharmacoepidemiologic designs described below.

There are some specific adverse events[7] that are known to be most frequently associated with, for instance biological drugs, such as autoimmune reactions, pure red blood cells aplasia (see case report # 7 in Chapter 4), Stevens–Johnson syndrome, progressive multifocal leukoencephalopathy (PML), and others.

Therefore, when these events are spontaneously reported, manufacturers should put more emphasis on these reports to promote fast and detailed follow-ups. They can also put in place an appropriate pharmacoepidemiologic design to further demonstrate whether a real causality link exists between the exposure to the health product and this specific adverse drug reaction.

2.5.3 Causality Assessment

A causality assessment is a method for assigning probability of causation to a suspected adverse drug reaction and the use of a health product. Analysis of causality consists of answering the question: *Is the factor A (health product A) the cause of the event B (e.g., anemia)*? In all cases, for causality to be true, it is pertinent that the exposure (to health product A) preceded the occurrence of the adverse event (anemia). Here anemia is just an example but any other adverse event could have been used for illustrative purposes.

Causality may be analyzed at the individual level by answering the following question: *Did the health product use in this study produce the event of anemia observed in this patient*? Or, at the population level by answering the following question: *Does the use of this health product increase the risk of developing anemia*?

A factor is called a "*specific relation*" if the occurrence of the event requires its presence (i.e., the factor will be found in all the subjects having presented the anemia, but its presence does not inevitably result in the occurrence of anemia).

On the other hand, a factor is called a "*sufficient relation*" if its presence inevitably causes anemia to happen (in which case all those exposed to this factor will present the anemia, although this does not necessarily mean that the factor will be found in all the subjects having presented the anemia).

Much more common (especially in pharmacoepidemiology) is the multifactorial causality in which several factors are identified as, independently or not, increasing the risk of the occurrence of the anemia, without any of them being specific or sufficient relations on their own.

In the strictest sense, only a controlled clinical trial with random allocation of treatment or exposure, and where a statistically significant association between exposure and the occurrence of an event is observed, can allow us to conclude to a causal relationship.

In observational epidemiology or pharmacoepidemiology studies (discuss in Chapter 3), the absence of a strong experimental design limits the validity of causal inference, notably because of the possible existence of bias and confounding factors.

As demonstrated in Chapter 4, case # 3, to assess the probability of an adverse drug reaction being related to a specific health product we use specific forms. Naranjo et al. created the Naranjo probability scale, which is made up of a series of 10 yes/no/do not know questions; each response is assigned a different value, and certain questions are assigned more points than others if the criteria are considered more important.

This produces a weighted score that the clinician can assign to the causality of each case as follows: unlikely (0), possible (1−4), probable (5−8), or certain (>9).[10]

2.5.4 Summary Reports

With the globalization of the drug industry and the withdrawal of some drugs from the market for safety reasons, regulatory authorities such as Health Canada, the FDA, the EMA, and others have recognized the need to better plan and implement earlier pharmacovigilance activities for adverse drug reactions, ideally before the authorization for marketing, and throughout the life cycle of health products.

To facilitate the work of the manufacturers, the International Conference on Harmonisation of Technical Requirements for Registration of Pharmaceuticals for Human Use (ICH) has developed various Guides and Guidelines that can be used by the manufacturers for the pharmacovigilance activities of adverse drug reactions in accordance with the Food and Drug Act and Regulations. For more information about these ICH Guidelines please follow this link: http://www.ich.org/products/guidelines/safety/article/safety-guidelines.html.

In accordance with article C.01.018 of the Food and Drug and Regulations (1) the manufacturer is to prepare a report that synthesizes information received regarding adverse drug reactions on an annual basis. The 12-month period covered by the annual report must be specified by the manufacturer (see the annex at the end of this book for a better discussion of the regulations surrounding the life cycle of health products including the summary reports).

In addition, according to article C.01.019 of the Food and Drug and Regulations, the Minister may, for the purposes of assessment of the safety and efficacy of the drug, request in writing that the manufacturer submits a summary report on a specific issue of concern, if one exists. In both cases, the summary report must be kept on site by the manufacturer or be easy to access and must, on request, be submitted to Health Canada (and other regulatory agencies) within a period of 30 calendar days following the request.

When Health Canada (and other regulatory agencies) requests the annual safety report from manufacturers, it can be requested in different forms depending on the needs of Health Canada (and other regulatory agencies), and it is best to present the report according to the format and standards set out in the ICH Guidelines for each of the following documents: Periodic Safety Update Reports (PSURs), Periodic Benefit-Risk Evaluation Reports (PBRER), Risk Management Plans (RMPs), and Development Safety Update Reports (DSURs). Each of these reports will be described in the sections that follow.

2.5.4.1 Periodic Safety Update Reports

The PSUR is a stand-alone document allowing for a periodic but complete assessment of data on the safety of a marketed health product. The format and content permit providing an evaluation of the benefit/risk ratio of a health product for submission by the marketing authorization holder at defined time points during the postauthorization phase.

The PSUR is also a safety summary on international data on a health product used to facilitate the postapproval marketing communication between the manufacturers and regulatory agencies such as Health Canada.

It reports adverse effects associated with taking a health product, observed over a period of 12 months, usually based on the health product's international birth date, in accordance with article C.01.018 of the Food and Drug Regulations (See Annex 3).

In addition, according to article C.01.019 of the Food and Drug Regulations, the PSUR may be requested by Health Canada (and other regulatory agencies) for a shorter period of time or as needed if a safety concern warrants the request. Also notice that these articles are not only limited to the PSUR but also apply to other summary reports (See Annex 1).

According to Klepper (2004), the PSUR is also an important source for the identification of new safety signals, a way to determine a change in the benefit/risk ratio, an effective way to communicate risks to regulators, and an indicator that signals the need to set up risk management measures. It is also a mechanism for the follow-up and assessment on the effectiveness of these measures.

For these reasons, the PSUR can be a very important tool in the pharmacovigilance of adverse drug reactions. However, this document is largely dependent on the quality of the available data. Despite the fact that it is gradually replaced by the Periodic Benefit-Risk Evaluation Report (PBRER), it is still used by many manufacturers and Health Canada (and other regulatory agencies) continues to review it.

2.5.4.1.1 Usefulness of the Periodic Safety Update Reports

The usefulness of this tool for the identification and prevention of adverse drug reactions has been recently verified by Ebbers et al.,[11] with a pharmacoepidemiologic study in the form of a cross-sectional analysis. The details on how to perform a cross-sectional study are presented below.

This cross-sectional analysis was performed on 70 PSURs submitted to the EMA between July 1, 2008 and June 30, 2010. Possible safety concerns have been observed in 57 (83%) of all surveyed PSUR. Of these, 26 (37%) led to changes at the level of the warnings section of the European Summary of Product Characteristics (SPC). In comparison with the new products, the products authorized for more than 10 years contained far fewer safety concerns (60% against 92%; $P < .01$) and required fewer changes to the SPC (15 against 46%; $P = .03$).

These authors also concluded from the pharmacoepidemiologic cross-sectional analysis that PSURs facilitate communication between regulators and manufacturers, regarding possible safety issues that arise during the course of a product's life cycle. Nevertheless, for long-term established products and evaluations from the PSUR rarely lead to regulatory action.

Bouvy et al.[12] recently analyzed the cost-effectiveness of all PSURs submitted for biological products in Europe between 1995 and 2009 by comparing two regulatory scenarios: the monitoring of the complete regulation (submit PSUR and other documents on the pharmacovigilance of adverse effects, including adverse drug reaction spontaneous reporting, postapproval safety studies, and the risk management plan).

The cost-effectiveness of the complete regulation monitoring (including the submission of PSUR) versus limited regulation (no submission of PSUR) was 342,110 euros per quality-adjusted life per year. This suggests that the use of this tool in the prevention of adverse drug reactions is cost-effective.[12]

2.5.4.2 Periodic Benefit-Risk Evaluation Report

As mentioned above, the main objective of the PSUR is to provide a periodic and complete safety profile based on what is currently known regarding the authorized health product. However, the information on the efficacy, the restrictions of use, the alternative treatments, and many other aspects of the health product therapy must also be considered in the assessment of the risks and benefits of health products. That is what the PBRER proposes. Given the fact that the assessment of the risk of a health product has its real significance when the product is also assessed in the light of its benefits; it can be added that the PBRER gives greater attention to the benefits (efficacy) than the PSUR.

2.5.4.2.1 The Periodic Benefit-Risk Evaluation Report Utility

Furlan[13] has considered the main safety features included in the various ICH Guidelines such as the PSUR, RMP, and DSUR (see below). He finds that the main elements and sources of information contained in these various guidelines overlap greatly with one another. What is to be considered in a context of limited resources?

The author proposes to reduce these overlaps as all these "regulatory" periodic reports should be in the form of a single document. This report should include all available information from all possible sources in regard to the identified and potential risks of a health product.

This single document should be updated on a regular (annual) basis or on request by Health Canada (and other regulatory agencies) to be in compliance with articles C.01.018 and C.01.019 of the Food and Drug Regulations (See Annex 1). One of the factors that led to the revision of the ICH E2C (R1) Guidelines is a desire to improve efficacy by reducing duplication of effort required for the preparation of the various regulatory documents.

Therefore, the guideline was drafted so that related sections of the PBRER, the DSUR, and the safety specifications of the RMP can be identical in terms of content. That being said, PBRER is still a very useful tool to generate hypotheses of an association between exposure to the health product and an adverse effect that are verifiable with one of the pharmacoepidemiologic study designs described in Chapter 3.

2.5.4.3 The Risk Management Plan

The RMP is a plan to perform activities relating to the detection, assessment, understanding, reporting, and prevention of adverse effects of health product during clinical trials. This plan should be initiated early and modified as necessary throughout the development process for a new health product in development for new indications.

The overall objective of the RMP is to ensure that the benefits of a particular health product (or a series of health products) exceed the risks by the greatest achievable margin for the individual patient and for the target population as a whole. This can be done either by increasing the benefits or by reducing the risks. The risk management has three stages that are interrelated and reiterative: (1) characterization of the safety profile of the health product including what is known and not known; (2) planning of pharmacovigilance activities to characterize risks and identify new risks and increase the knowledge in general about the safety profile of the health product; (3) planning and implementation of risk minimization and mitigation and assessment of the effectiveness of these activities.

Carefully planned, the adverse drug reactions throughout the pharmacovigilance activities can reduce the health product risk of toxicity and increase the benefits to patients. For more information on the content and format requirements of the RMP and to consult the ICH E2E Guidelines, visit the following link: http://www.ich.org/fileadmin/Public_Web_Site/ICH_Products/Guidelines/Efficacy/E2E/Step4/E2E_Guideline.pdf.

This guideline is also implemented for the planning of adverse drug reaction prevention activities during the postapproval marketing period. It also sets out the principles of good clinical practices for the design and implementation of postmarketing pharmacoepidemiologic studies including phase IV studies. The guideline is composed of three main components: (1) the pharmacovigilance specifications; (2) the pharmacovigilance plan; (3) the start-up of the postauthorization safety pharmacoepidemiologic studies.

In brief, the RMP is a very important tool in the assessment of the benefit/risk ratio and in the prevention of adverse drug reactions throughout the life cycle of health products. Even if presented differently, these main components are the elements that should be included in the other summary reports mentioned here.

2.5.4.3.1 The Risk Minimization Activities (Measures)

An intervention intended to prevent or reduce the probability of the occurrence of an adverse reaction associated with the exposure to a health product, or to reduce its severity should it occur. These activities may consist of routine risk minimization (e.g., product information) or additional risk-minimization activities (e.g., health-care professional add letters or patient communications/educational materials).

2.5.4.3.2 Pharmacovigilance Specifications

This part of an RMP provides a synopsis of the safety profile of the health product(s) and should include what is known and not known about the health product(s). It should be a summary of the important identified risks of a health product, important potential risks, and missing information. It should also address the populations potentially at risk (where the health product is likely to be used, i.e., both labeled and off-labeled use), and outstanding safety questions that warrant further investigation to refine understanding of the risk—benefit ratio during the postauthorization period.

The specification may include, but is not limited to (1) identify the preclinical phase safety concerns; (2) analyze the missing preclinical data; (3) assess adverse drug reactions observed during the clinical trials; (4) analyze human safety databases and the frequency of adverse drug reactions that have been detected during these clinical trials; (5) analyze potential adverse drug reactions that require a more thorough assessment throughout pharmacoepidemiologic studies to clarify the assumptions of risk; (6) assess populations that have not been studied in the preauthorization phase via pharmacoepidemiologic studies; (7) analyze documented drug interactions; (8) determine the potential for unidentified interactions that may occur during the postmarketing approval; (9) carry out epidemiological studies of diseases; (10) assess the effects of drug class.

As for the other safety summary reports, the RMP is a very useful tool to generate hypotheses of an association between exposure to a drug and an adverse effect that can be verified with various pharmacoepidemiologic study designs described in Chapter 3 with concrete examples in Chapter 4.

These specifications will help the manufacturers and the regulatory agencies to identify all specific data that need to be collected and analyzed during the postmarketing period. This also facilitates the preparation of the adverse drug reactions pharmacovigilance plan that incorporates the concept of life cycle of health products. For more information on the content and format requirements of the RMP and to consult the ICH E2E Guidelines, visit the following link: http://www.ich.org/fileadmin/Public_Web_Site/ICH_Products/Guidelines/Efficacy/E2E/Step4/E2E_Guideline.pdf.

2.5.4.3.3 Usefulness of Risk Management Plan

To determine if the RMP is an effective tool to improve the safety of drugs, Frau et al. conducted a pharmacoepidemiologic study designed to describe the characteristics of these plans for 15 drugs approved by the EMA and their impact on the postapproval pharmacovigilance period. Among 90 new chemical entities approved during 2006 and 2007, 15 were selected and their security and their RMP components have been analyzed.

All safety pharmacovigilance communications related to these drugs in the postmarketing period were also considered. A total of 157 safety specifications have been implemented for these evaluated drugs. Postmarket safety concerns have emerged for 12 of them, leading to 39 changes to the Summary of Product Characteristics (SPC) of these European products. Nearly half of these changes, 19 (49%), covered security features not provided by the RMP. In addition, 9 safety communications have been published for 6 of the 15 drugs evaluated.

The pharmacoepidemiologic study revealed that the RMP is an effective tool to prevent adverse effects associated with drugs, but several activities offered by the RMPs do not seem to be sufficient to deal with all the potential risks associated with drugs.

The authors add that the lack of risk communication between clinicians and the public and especially the limited risk assessing transparency seems to transform the RMP into a tool to reassure the public when a drug has been insufficiently evaluated and received a marketing authorization prematurely.[14]

2.5.4.4 Development Safety Update Report

The DSUR is a periodic summary of safety information for regulators, including any changes in the benefit–risk relationship, for a drug, biologic, or vaccine under development, prepared by the sponsor for all its clinical trials.

During the clinical development, periodic safety analysis is crucial to the ongoing risk assessment of participants in clinical trials for all marketed or nonmarketed drugs at all dosage forms, for all indications and for all patient populations in study with the health product used. Whereas the majority of clinical trials are multinational and/or multicenter, it is necessary that these reporting requirements be harmonized for all regulatory authorities around the world including Health Canada, which adopted this report in June 2012.

The concept of DSUR was first introduced by the Council for International Organizations of Medical Sciences (CIOMS) VI working group (http://www.cioms.ch/) and pursued by the CIOMS VII Working Group. In 2010, the ICH published the E2F Guidelines on the DSUR, incorporating the context, objectives, and the scope of the DSUR by providing advice on its content.

For more information on the content and format requirements of the DSUR, the readers can consult the ICH E2F Guidelines and visit the following link: http://www.ich.org/fileadmin/Public_Web_Site/ICH_Products/Guidelines/Efficacy/E2F/Step4/E2F_Step_4.pdf.

2.5.4.4.1 Usefulness of the Development Safety Update Report

The main objective of the DSUR is to present a comprehensive annual review of the safety information associated with a drug in development collected during the reporting period.

The DSUR's unique value is to identify the trends and characteristics of the safety issues related to a drug in development, which cannot be obtained by looking at the individual case reports in isolation. It is therefore a tool for the prevention of the adverse effects associated with the very important drugs, serving not only in the analysis of safety signals but also to update the product monograph (when the product is marketed) and to update the Investigator's Brochure (when the product is in the research phase).

The DSUR allows for an assessment of the health product within the life cycle concept including the safety of participants in clinical trials and, in many cases, the safety of patients in real-life (in postmarketing approval) condition.

2.6 ACTIVE SURVEILLANCE (PHARMACOVIGILANCE)

Active surveillance, unlike passive surveillance, seeks to determine potential safety concerns through a continuous preorganized assessment process as completely as possible. It involves regular systematic collection of clinical information on a population of patients who receive drugs that are on the market.

There are several ways by which this clinical information may be collected: sentinel sites, intensive monitoring protocols, follow-up of specific events, patients' registries, observational studies, clinical trials, and others. For more information on this collecting of information methods, please consult Chapter 4 and the glossary of terms in Annex 2.

In general, it is easier to get comprehensive evaluation of adverse drug reactions through an active surveillance system compared to a passive reporting system. In the following pages, we will discuss on patients registries emphasizing on the most important tools of the active pharmacovigilance system, which are the pharmacoepidemiologic studies.

2.6.1 Patient Registries

A patient registry is a list of patients presenting with the same characteristic(s). This characteristic can be a disease (disease registry) or a specific exposure (drug registry). Both types of registries, which only differ by the type of patient data of interest, can collect a wide variety of information using standardized questionnaires in a prospective fashion. Exposure (drug) registries collect information over time on populations exposed to health products of interest and/or specific populations. Patients can be included in a cohort study to collect data on adverse events using standardized questionnaires. They can be useful for signal detection, particularly of rare outcomes.

In many countries, disease-based registers have been established for the specific reporting of clinical information and management of certain diseases and procedures. The potential for analyzing the effects and safety of drugs has further developed with the introduction of electronic health records containing not only prescription drug data but also other clinical parameters, such as diagnosis, vital signs, laboratory data, and more or less structured clinical notes. In some countries, biobanks have also been established enabling linking drug utilization to genetic data.

At the market-authorization phase, all the risks and all the adverse effects related to a health product are rarely entirely known.[15] This section is therefore intended to describe the essential role of patient registries in the active surveillance of specialized health products. Thus, patient registries have become more attractive in the active surveillance of adverse drug reactions. For more information on the use of patients registries in the active surveillance of health products, please consult Chapter 4 for concrete examples.

However, their exact role continues to evolve. These registries consist of a defined patient population with the same characteristics for which data are collected in a systematic way over a defined period of time. Therefore, they are useful for providing reliable estimates of the adverse events incidence among a defined population and they are also very useful for pharmacoepidemiologic studies.[15]

The purpose of these registries is to improve our knowledge on the safety of a health product, especially on the long-term use of this product.[8]

However, as registries do not systematically include control groups of similar patients who did not receive the health product, they are not able to answer questions related to the efficacy or treatment effect and cannot serve as replacements for clinical trials. In addition, due to their high operational costs, registries are more important for monitoring highly specialized health products that are used in significant clinical settings.[15]

The disease registries, such as registries for blood dyscrasias, severe skin reactions, congenital, or other abnormalities can help collect pharmacoepidemiologic data on drug exposure and other factors associated with a particular clinical condition. A disease registry can also be used as data for a case-control study (see below) comparing exposure to the drug (cases) identified in the registry and a selected group of patients in the registry with another condition, or from patients outside the registry (controls).[15]

The drug or exposure registries are used in populations exposed to specific health products (for example, the rheumatoid arthritis registry in patients exposed to biological therapies) to determine if a drug has a specific effect in this group of patients.[15]

Certain exposure registries address exposures to drugs in specific populations, such as pregnant women. With this registry, patients can be monitored over time and included in a cohort study to collect data on adverse events using standardized questionnaires.[15]

These cohort studies (see below in Chapter 3) can be used to measure the impact, but, without a comparison group cannot provide proof of an association (causality) between the adverse events and the health product. However, they can be useful to increase signal detection in particular for rare adverse events. This type of registry can be very useful during the safety review of an orphan drug, indicated for a specific rare condition, for example. For more information, please consult Chapter 4 for concrete examples.

One of the most important and known examples of exposure registry involved natalizumab, which is a specific monoclonal antibody for the $\alpha 4$ integrin that is used for the treatment of multiple sclerosis.

Clinical trials and postmarketing data indicated that natalizumab is associated with an increased risk of PML, a potentially fatal disease affecting the central nervous system.

Natalizumab was voluntarily withdrawn from the market by the manufacturer in 2005, when the initial cases of PML associated with the use of natalizumab were identified.[8]

After a review of the safety and benefits of this biologic product, natalizumab was reintroduced on the market in 2006 under a risk-minimizing program for PML while patients receiving the drug are recorded and monitored for this specific adverse effect. The TYGRIS Registry aims to recruit 6000 patients worldwide; and follow-up of this registry will help to increase our knowledge about the security of this biologic product.[8]

There are other registries such as registries of specific conditions that include those put in place to monitor the treatment of rare diseases. The purpose of these registries is to identify the impact of different treatments in the long term. Clinical trials of drugs for these diseases are usually performed on just a few patients. Therefore, the safety information may be limited.

For example, the idursulphase is a health product used in the treatment of the Hunter syndrome, a rare genetic disease that occurs in approximately two people per million inhabitants. After the marketing authorization of the product, the manufacturer has implemented a registry called "Hunter Investigation" where all patients with the Hunter syndrome are invited to participate in the survey, regardless whether or not they are treated with idursulphase.

This registry will help provide information on the progress of the Hunter syndrome, as well as its associated medical consequences.[8] Even if often limited by the lack of a control group and the need to produce a comprehensive analysis of individual cases to maintain the data integrity, registries are useful for monitoring highly specialized drugs and rare health conditions.[15] They are also very useful to generate hypothesis for pharmacoepidemiologic studies.

2.7 CONCLUSIONS

The assessment and analysis of adverse drug reactions is critical for early detection of the potential security issues with health products. An effective assessment of these adverse effects either in pre- or in postapproval development market may point to the need to put in place additional security measures that can lead to a faster response by the regulatory agencies and the medical profession such as placing restrictions of use on some health products or in extreme cases, suspend the use of a health product.[16]

Historically, the premarket phase was the only phase for determination of effectiveness and safety of health products. The postapproval surveillance setting becomes more and more important in this environment; so we are now more talking to an assessment of the risks and benefits throughout the life cycle of a health product.

As it has been discussed in this chapter, there are important limitations to pharmacovigilance including the quality of the adverse drug reactions reporting, the absence of reporting, and others. However, the pharmacovigilance activities remain an essential discipline in the management of adverse effects of health products that are evolving.

Pharmacovigilance activities are essential to answer the safety questions posed by a number of more effective health products having inevitable and sometimes unpredictable potential to generate adverse effects.

Whether at the pre- or postapproval marketing level when adverse effects appear, it is essential that they are analyzed and reported through effective means to regulatory organizations to interpret their impacts (see Annex 1 for some regulations regarding the reporting of adverse drug reactions).

This chapter gives an overview of the main pharmacovigilance elements to be considered in the analysis and management of adverse drug reactions. Some of these elements will be explored in greater detail in the chapters that follow. The reader is invited to consult Annex 1 at the end of this book to help consolidate the information that has been provided so far.

REFERENCES

1. World Health Organization. *Pharmacovigilance: ensuring the safe use of medicines*; 2004. http://apps.who.int/iris/handle/10665/68782.
2. Eurasanté. *Entreprendre et Réussir.* La Pharmacovigilance; 2006, 39P.
3. Health Product Vigilance Framework; 2012. Disponible à https://www.canada.ca/en/health-canada/services/drugs-health-products/reports-publications/medeffect-canada/health-product-vigilance-framework-health-canada-2012.html.
4. Dugair M. *Le programme Canadien de Pharmacovigilance: Peut-on prévenir de nouveaux cas Vioxx?* Cahier de Formation Continue de l'Actualité Pharmaceutique; 2009:1–4.
5. Yates N, Lee DK, Maher M. Health Canada's progressive licensing framework. *CMAJ.* 2007;176:1845–1847.
6. Maher M. Legislative and regulatory modernization for therapeutic products. *J Popul Ther Clin Pharmacol.* 2010;17:E341–E348.
7. Talbot J, Nilson B. Pharmacovigilance in pharmaceutical industry. *Br J Clin Pharmacol.* 1998;45:427–431.
8. Wise L, Parkinson J, Raine J, Breckenridge A. New approaches to drug safety: a pharmacovigilance tool kit. *Nat Rev Drug Discov.* 2009;8:779–782.
9. Jacob D, Marrón B, Ehrlich J, Rutherford PA. Pharmacovigilance as a tool for safety and monitoring: a review of general issues and the specific challenges with end-stage renal failure patients. *Drug, Healthc and Patient Saf.* 2013;5:105–112.
10. Naranjo CA, Busto U, Sellers EM, et al. A method for estimating the probability of adverse drug reactions. *Clin Pharmacol Ther.* 1981;30:239–245.
11. Ebbers HC, Al-Temimi E, Moors EH, et al. Differences between post-authorization adverse drug reactions of biopharmaceuticals and small molecules. *BioDrugs.* 2013;27:167–174.
12. Bouvy JC, Ebbers HC, Schellenkens H, Koopmanschap MA. The cost-effectiveness of periodic safety update reports for biologicals in Europe. *Clin Pharmacol Ther.* 2013;93:433–442.
13. Furlan G. Using resources for scientific-driven pharmacovigilance: from many product safety documents to one product safety master file: current opinion. *Drug Saf.* 2012;35:615–622.

14. Frau S, Pous MF, Luppino MR, Conforti A. Risk Management Plans: are they a tool for improving drug safety? *Eur J Clin Pharmacol.* 2010;66:785–790.
15. Willis CD, McNeil JJ, Cameron PA, Phillips LE. Monitoring Drug Safety with registries: useful components of postmarketing pharmacovigilance systems. *J Clin Epidemiol.* 2012;65:121–125.
16. Lemmens T, Gibson S. Decreasing the data deficit: improving post-market surveillance in pharmaceutical regulations. *McGill L J.* 2014;59(4):944–989.

Chapter 3

Pharmacoepidemiology in the Prevention of Adverse Drug Reactions

3.1 INTRODUCTION

As briefly stated in the introduction, pharmacoepidemiology refers to the study of interactions between health products and populations. More specifically, "*pharmacoepidemiology*" can be defined as the study of the therapeutic effect(s), risks, and uses of health products, usually in large populations, using epidemiological methods.

Although experimental studies may be preferred for establishing the efficacy of a drug, the goal of the pharmacoepidemiology approach is generally to describe the situation in real life, avoiding, as much as possible, any modification to this situation caused by the study itself. Pharmacoepidemiology applies to descriptive approaches (e.g., describing a phenomenon or estimating a risk in real circumstances) as well as to etiologic approaches (e.g., determining the extent to which a health product is likely to increase a risk under real conditions of use). For those interested, we have created a glossary of terms related to pharmacoepidemiology and its associated components to summarize the information presented here (see Annex 2).

3.2 PRODUCT LIFE CYCLE

Epidemiologic methods have become increasingly recognized as a valuable tool for better characterizing the benefit–risk profile throughout all stages of the product life cycle. During the preauthorization phase, pharmacoepidemiologic studies are useful for determining the background incidence and/or prevalence rate (see Annex 2) of a specific disease within a target population. This information can then be used by the sponsor to provide a rationale to justify the clinical development of a new health product and if the benefit/risk ratio is positive, to further justify the approval of the new health product under development.

Pharmacoepidemiology and Pharmacovigilance. https://doi.org/10.1016/B978-0-12-816183-8.00003-2

These background rates of adverse events in the target population can be identified to complement data obtained from clinical trials, which would allow for more meaningful safety assessments. For example, the rate of specific adverse events in the target population identified during the premarket phase III clinical trials for a new health product can be compared with the rate of adverse events observed in the general population, which can be used for establishing the benefit/risk ratio of the new health product.

Then these adverse event signals can also be followed with postmarket surveillance activities (see Fig. 1.1 of Chapter 1) to allow for a more meaningful assessment of the safety profile of a health product throughout its life cycle.

Pharmacoepidemiologic studies can used for both passive and active surveillance of drug safety. Even before a new health product is authorized for use, important risk factors in patients who will take this health product can be identified using pharmacoepidemiologic studies. This is particularly relevant to the prescriber because the decision whether or not to give this new health product to a particular patient will depend on whether their patients has the identified risks factors.[1]

Similarly, the information found from pharmacoepidemiologic studies prior to market authorization of a new health product cam be included in the product monograph to inform the prescribers and the patients about specific contraindications, warnings/precautions, drug interactions, etc., which appear to be associated with the new health product based on the analysis of the patients populations that were studied.

Finally, after the product has been authorized for distribution to the public, pharmacoepidemiologic studies, referred to as phase IV studies (see Annex 2), may be requested by the regulatory agency to follow the concerns identified before the authorization of the health product and/or to identify potential new safety risks associated with the health product throughout its life cycle.

Of course, the scenarios described here are only a few examples of the type of information epidemiology studies can provide to supplement the data obtained from more rigorous clinical trial during the premarket phase of a product's life cycle.

3.3 THE NECESSITY OF PHARMACOEPIDEMIOLOGY

The drug approval process for new products authorized in Canada, and elsewhere, essentially involves a comprehensive analysis of nonclinical and clinical studies. However, the management of adverse effects associated with these new health products does not end on granting market authorization. Rather, these surveillance activities continue throughout the entire drug's life cycle and this is made possible essentially through the passive and active surveillance of adverse drug reactions in the postmarket setting. As mentioned in Chapter 2, passive or active surveillance of adverse drug reactions includes pharmacoepidemiologic studies.[2]

Pharmacoepidemiologic studies can be used to identify unexpected or rare safety issues and detect changes in frequency of expected adverse events, and this leads to the reevaluation of a product's benefit–risk ratio. Postmarket research is important for the industry because they can use this data to submit future amendments to the approved indications for their products and demonstrate the safety and effectiveness of their products, especially compared to others. Postmarket drug research is especially an important tool for regulatory agencies and the physicians/patients using the products. When a regulator grants authorization for a drug, it is largely a result of the data obtained from randomized clinical trials (RCTs).

These RCTs are designed with the purpose of demonstrating efficacy (not safety): smaller sample sizes are used, length of follow-up is short, and strict inclusion/exclusion criteria are used.[3–5]

A smaller sample size means the study will not have enough power to detect small changes in frequency for commonly reported adverse events or to detect rare, but serious, adverse drug reactions. A short follow-up period means that serious adverse reactions may not be identified because they do not develop immediately. A strict inclusion/exclusion criteria means the population used in the study is likely healthier, excludes children, elderly and pregnant or breast feeding women, uses no/limited concomitant medications, and has a less complicated medical history than the general population that will actually end up using the medication. These criteria are made restrictive to increase the internal validity of the results to produce an accurate and unbiased estimate of efficacy. However, the trade-off is that RCTs have low external validity; this means the results cannot be generalized to the heterogeneous population that will actually end up using the drug including patients with several concomitant medications, complex medical histories, and increased severity of illness and pregnant women, children, and the elderly.[3–5] The safety profile might then change once the drug is approved, which may require a reevaluation of the benefit–risk profile for the product.

Thus, there is a clear need for high-quality pharmacoepidemiology research in the postmarket setting for the timely identification of any significant safety issues that arise when used in the real world (i.e., uncontrolled setting) to protect the health of patients.

3.4 TOOLS IN PHARMACOEPIDEMIOLOGY

It is important to have a good understanding of the various tools available to perform the appropriate pharmacoepidemiologic studies for the appropriate situation and context. Even more important is that we should have a clear understanding of the strengths and limits of each of these study designs. These strengths and limits are further illustrated by concrete examples in the case reports provided in Chapter 4.

There is no gold standard when it comes to study design in pharmacoepidemiology because each of design has its own strengths and weaknesses. Therefore, the choice of the study design is decided according to what will work best to answer the particular research question involved.

There are also other important considerations, such as the availability of data, the constraints of time, the cost and the feasibility, and several other important factors that should also be considered when determining the most appropriate study design for a particular situation. In all cases, the methodology used should always be supported by appropriate scientific/clinical rationale.

In the subsections that follow you will find a discussion regarding the available tools used for pharmacoepidemiologic research. First, at the forefront of routine pharmacovigilance, we will discuss the continuous monitoring of spontaneously reported adverse events. Then, we will discuss traditional epidemiology observational study designs, which can be used to study specific associations between drug(s) and adverse or benefits events or other safety issues using quantifiable measures of association/risk. We will also review the designs for advanced studies.

For concrete examples on the use of these designs, please also consult the case reports provided in Chapter 4.

3.4.1 Adverse Reactions Spontaneously Reported

As discussed above in Chapter 2, the analysis of spontaneously reported adverse events is at the front line of postmarket drug safety surveillance. A case report describes the occurrence of an unusual/unexpected adverse event that health-care professionals/patients suspect to be related to a particular health product/intervention (see Annex 2).[6] Drug companies are usually required to report adverse events to regulatory authorities such as Health Canada, the FDA, the European Medicines Agency (EMA), and others.

Similar to a case report, a case series provides a detailed account of a group of similar patients (instead of only one individual) to describe the occurrence of an unusual adverse event/experience that occurred after taking the same health product.[6] When reviewing case reports/series, the objective is to determine the likelihood that the exposure to the drug (or something else) was associated with the occurrence of the reported adverse event.

The clinical/medical evaluation of such reports may lead to the early identification of a serious unexpected adverse drug reaction caused by a specific health product. This could result in a product recall, issuance of health-care professional and public communication notices, and/or changes in labeling. Additional details are provided in Chapter 4, including concrete examples of actions that regulatory agencies can put in place to ensure the safety of clinical trial participants, as well as the safety of patients in the real world (i.e., uncontrolled postmarket setting) according to the principles of the therapeutic product life cycle (see Fig. 1.1 of Chapter 1).

Unfortunately, however, determining causality from case reports or case series data is often challenging. This is mainly because case reports are often poorly documented and do not include important details related to the exposure and/or the outcome. For example, details regarding dosage, duration, and timing of the exposure are often omitted. As well, the details regarding outcomes such as severity of the event, medical confirmation with laboratory tests, or whether the outcome resolved or not after stopping the health product are not provided (see Annex 2).

Furthermore, other alternative explanations for the adverse event such as the patient's medical history, the use of concomitant medications, or certain lifestyle risk factors are not reported.

Without knowing the aforementioned details, an accurate causality assessment is almost impossible in these situations.

The reporting of such adverse events may also be biased. Because spontaneously reported adverse events are reported voluntarily, there may be a bias with regard to how or when a physician or patient submits a case report (see Annex 2).

Under-reporting of adverse events is also an issue: some estimates have been made suggesting that the FDA receives only between 8% and 13%[7] of all serious adverse events, whereas in another study they estimate this number to be less than 1%.[8]

Nonetheless, the analysis of case reports and case series data remains an important component of postmarket drug passive surveillance. In fact, there have been cases where correctly and spontaneously reported adverse events have led to the identification of important safety issues for certain therapeutic products. For example, postmarketing case reports of myocarditis following clozapine exposure led to an FDA-requested update in the product's black box warning of the product monograph for this health product (see Chapter 4 for concrete examples of this situation).

More serious consequences have also occurred, such as the withdrawal of Lotronex from the market following reported cases of ischemic colitis following drug exposure.[5]

Below, we describe a variety of techniques that can be used to analyze adverse events reported spontaneously, either qualitatively or quantitatively. Qualitative and quantitative methods should be used to supplement one another and are not a substitution for one another.

3.4.1.1 Qualitative Detection of Signals

Traditionally, clinicians perform a qualitative analysis of the information provided in each case report individually and make a judgment regarding causality based on their clinical expertise on a case-by-case basis. This type of analysis is unstructured and subjective.

Therefore attempts have been made to develop a list of important common criteria for determining causality to be used by all clinicians. The common criteria (such as temporal sequence, dechallenge/rechallenge, and confounding factors) allow clinicians to qualitatively assign each case as either not related, unlikely related, possibly related, probably related, or definitely related (see Table 3.1 for a definition of these terms).[9,10]

TABLE 3.1 Causality Assessment Descriptions

Not related/unrelated	This suggests that there is no causal association between the investigational product and the reported event.
Unlikely related	This suggests that the clinical picture is highly consistent with a cause other than the investigational product, but attribution cannot be made with absolute certainty and a relationship between the investigational product and adverse event cannot be excluded with complete confidence.
Possibly related	This suggests that treatment with the investigational product may have caused or contributed to the adverse event (i.e., the event follows a reasonable temporal sequence from the time of drug administration and/or follows a known response pattern to the investigational product but could also have been produced by other factors).
Probably related	This suggests that a reasonable temporal sequence of the event with the investigational product administration exists and also the likely causal association of the event with the investigational product. This will be based on the known pharmacological action of the investigational product, known or previously reported adverse reactions to the investigational product or class of drugs, or judgment based on the investigator's clinical experience.
Definitely related	This temporal relationship to the investigational product, other conditions (concurrent illness, concurrent medication reaction, or progression/ expression of disease state) do not appear to explain the adverse event, corresponds with the known pharmaceutical profile, improvement on discontinuation, reappearance, on rechallenge.

For more information about these definitions, please consult the ICH-E2A at the link provided at the end of this book.

One such example is the World Health Organization Uppsala Monitoring Center (WHO-UMC) Standardized Case Causality Assessment criteria (see: http://www.who.int/medicines/areas/quality_safety/safety_efficacy/WHO causality_assessment.pdf).

Alternatively, several algorithms have also been published to improve the causality assessment process by calculating a weighted score based on a set of criteria. However, a universally accepted method among all these still does not exist.[9,10]

In 1991, Naranjo et al. developed a method to assess the probability of an adverse drug reaction being related to a specific health product.

A study that compared the WHO-UMC criteria and the Naranjo algorithm found a disagreement in causality assessment in 45 out of 913 case reports analyzed (4.9%) and also found that the WHO-UMC criteria was less time-consuming than the Naranjo algorithm.[9] Both methods continue to be commonly used today.

For further information on performing causality assessment, please consult Chapter 4.

Regardless of which qualitative method is used, however, the validity of each assessment is largely dependent on the quality of the information reported in the case report. When several important data are missing, as mentioned above, the causality will be impossible to determine.

Furthermore, given the high volume of spontaneous adverse events and adverse reaction reports there is simply a lack of adequate resources to conduct a clinical evaluation of each individual case report.

Even if the timely clinically review of each case report was possible, it would be hard to capture all types of trends and patterns presenting in the data.

To overcome some of these challenges, data mining using quantitative methods to automatically detect safety signals from large databases of reported adverse events can be used.

However, the increasing amount of data does not imply that studies have become easier to conduct. In many databases, data input remains incomplete and, therefore, there is the potential for bias. Furthermore, health-care data are difficult to analyze due to the large number of variables and the interrelated nature of these variables. In the section that follows, we will discuss quantitative detection of safety signals.

3.4.1.2 Quantitative Detection of Signals

Data mining in the context of pharmacovigilance refers to the act of searching through existing databases or other sources of spontaneously reported suspected adverse drug reactions to detect the presence and determine the strength of safety signals using disproportionality analysis.[11] For more concrete examples on the use of this quantitative detection of signals, please take a close look at some of the case reports provided in Chapter 4.

Disproportionality analysis quantifies the degree of unexpectedness of a specific drug-adverse event combination. The combination is considered disproportional when the association is higher than expected.[12]

As mentioned earlier, spontaneously reported adverse event databases are generated from voluntary reporting by health-care professionals and/or patients. Drug companies also have their own databases for collecting data from both clinical trial and commercial sources.

Routine pharmacovigilance activities, now commonly include the implementation of automatic mathematical algorithms that trigger potential safety signals when the level of disproportionality exceeds a certain predefined threshold.

There are two approaches that can be used for disproportionality analysis: the "frequentist" approach, which relies on frequency of reported adverse event data, or the "Bayesian" approach that utilizes Bayesian probability theories to estimate disproportionality (see Glossary of terms at the end of this chapter).

The proportional reporting ratio (PRR) and the reporting odds ratio (ROR) are commonly used "frequentist" measures, whereas the Bayesian confidence propagation neural network (BCPNN) and the multi-item gamma Poisson shrinker (MGPS) are commonly used "Bayesian" measures.[12,13] In this section, we will provide a brief introduction to these four measures of disproportionality. The 2x2 contingency shown in Table 3.2 below will help to better understand how the PRR and ROR are calculated.

3.4.1.2.1 The Proportional Reporting Ratio

The PRR compares the proportion of an adverse event-drug combination among all people exposed to the drug with the proportion of the same adverse event–drug combination among people exposed to the other drugs in the

TABLE 3.2 2 × 2 Contingency Table Used for Disproportionality Analysis (Frequentist Approach)

	Case Reported adverse event (AE) of Interest	Case Did Not Report adverse event (AE) of Interest
Cases related to drug of interest	a	b
All other cases	c	d

Proportional reporting ratio (PRR) = [a/(a+b)]/[c/(c + d)]. Reporting odds ratio (ROR) = [a/b]/[c/d] = [a * d]/[b * c].

database.[14] Using the PRR method, a signal (see Annex 2) is detected when the three following conditions are met:

1. at least three cases of the specific adverse event–drug combination have been reported,
2. a PRR of at least 2,
3. chi-squared PRR of at least 4.

Notice that the chi-square test is a statistical test that determines whether an association is statistically significant. Alternatively 95% confidence intervals (see Annex 2) could also be calculated to test for statistical significance.[15]

The PRR is advantageous because it is a simple calculation that can be easily interpreted and used for the timely rapid identification of specific drug–event combinations that represent potential safety signals. The PRR does not require external data such as dispensed prescriptions or sales data to be used as a denominator for calculating a reporting rate. The PRR also is not affected by underreporting of adverse events, which is one of the major issues related to analyzing spontaneously reported data, provided that the magnitude of underreporting is similar across all adverse events (see Annex 2).[14]

However, if a specific drug–event combination is very common, the PRR is limited in that detecting other signals for that drug may become more difficult because the value of "b" would become larger, thereby decreasing the value of the numerator used in the PRR calculation, which will shrink the PRR. Alternatively an underestimated PRR can also be produced if a specific drug–event combination is common among an entire class of drugs.[15] One approach in dealing with these limitations is to remove the cases from the analysis that are responsible for masking the true PRR (see Annex 2).

3.4.1.2.2 The Reporting Odds Ratio

Using the same data, but thinking of the database as a case-control study, the ROR can alternatively be calculated as shown in the equation under Table 3.2. The advantages of the ROR are that it can be easily applied, and logistic regression analysis can be used to adjust for covariates and test for significant interaction terms (i.e., to investigate specific drug–drug interactions in relation to a reported adverse event).

Furthermore, the ROR is not sensitive to nonselective underreporting of a drug or adverse drug reactions. The disadvantage of the ROR is that it requires cells a, b, c, and d to all contain at least one report, which may not be the case for certain rare adverse drug reactions. In the event that only small numbers are reported in the cells a, b, c, and d, the ROR becomes a less-reliable estimate. Lastly, the interpretation of the ROR is not easily interpreted unlike the PRR that is more intuitive.[14]

3.4.1.2.3 Bayesian Approach

Unlike the "frequentist" approach, which relies solely on the frequency of the data reported in adverse event databases, the Bayesian approach uses measures of probability to detect potential safety signals (see Annex 2). The prior probability estimated reflects the probability of a specific adverse event–drug combination reported, assuming they are not associated with one another.

As case reports accumulate and if the specific drug–event combination is in fact reported more frequently, then the probability distribution changes. This is called the posterior probability (see Annex 2). When the posterior probability exceeds the prior probability, a potential safety signal is generated.

The BCPNN identifies signals using the probability distributions determined by the Information Component (see Annex 2).

The MGPS estimates the probability distributions using the empirical Bayes geometric mean. The calculations for these methods are complex and beyond the scope of this chapter, but detailed explanations have been provided elsewhere.[16–20]

The disadvantage of the Bayesian approach is that it is not transparent, which means individuals unfamiliar with Bayesian statistics will not easily be able to understand how signals are generated. Nonetheless, they are especially useful for identifying more complex patterns of adverse event reporting in databases, including higher-order combinations involving drug–drug interactions.[21]

Several studies have been performed to compare these four different quantitative signal detection methods.[17,22] Most studies show that all four methods produce roughly similar results, especially when the frequency of reported adverse event–drug combinations is higher.

However, when the reporting is very low, some slight differences may appear. In any case, each method has its own advantages and disadvantages, thus the decision to use a specific approach should be based on one's specific needs.[17] For example, WHO uses the BCPNN,[19] the FDA uses the MGPS,[20] and the EMA relies on the PRR.[23]

Regardless of the method used, the biases inherent in spontaneous adverse drug reaction reporting (voluntary reporting/underreporting and others) still exist (see Annex 2). Furthermore, these methods do not indicate causal associations; they only show mathematical associations.

As such, when a potential safety signal is identified, an expert clinician should always follow-up with a qualitative review of the case reports that report the specific adverse event–drug combination. It is imperative to consider that the qualitative and quantitative methods are meant to complement one another and not to replace one another. To help the readers better understand these important concepts, see the case report # 7 and others presented in Chapter 4.

3.4.2 Observational Study Designs Used in Pharmacoepidemiologic Research

As mentioned above, although the passive and active monitoring of reported adverse events is at the forefront of routine pharmacovigilance, they are not the only providers of safety information in the postmarket arena.

As discussed, it is often difficult to make a meaningful causality assessment due to the lack of adequately reported data included in these summary reports. Furthermore, even when possible associations between a drug and event are identified, further evidence is required to better characterize the strength of the association.

Traditional epidemiologic observational studies, on the other hand, can be used to study specific associations between drug(s) and adverse events, other safety issues, or even beneficial events, and they allow the researcher to produce a quantifiable measures of association and/or risk.

An observational study can be initiated to confirm or reject a hypothesis regarding an association between a specific drug and adverse event that was initially triggered by case reports or case series data. Alternatively, an observational study can also be planned ahead of time, for example when a product receives market authorization, to prospectively assess the safety and effectiveness of a drug once used in a noninterventional setting (i.e., in the real world).

These types of studies could be suggested, for example by a drug company, or planned at the request of a regulatory agency that feels the safety profile of the drug needs to be studied more closely. Observational studies can also be used for descriptive purposes to describe the burden of diseases in a population or as a drug utilization study to monitor patterns of use in target populations (see Annex 2).

Whether you are a scientific regulatory evaluator, a health-care provider, an academic researcher, or a member of the pharmaceutical health product industry, it is important to have a clear understanding of the different study designs available for pharmacoepidemiologic research and of the different measures that can be calculated to quantify the findings from pharmacoepidemiologic studies.

Also important is the ability to identify the strengths and limitations of each major study design and subsequently apply this knowledge to determine which of the study designs would be the most appropriate in a particular situation. The caveat is that there is no golden standard as to which study design is preferred for a specific scenario (see Annex 2).

The choice of study design is thus a matter of which approach best suits the research question. This entails a thoughtful consideration of which drug is being investigated, the nature of the adverse event/safety issue being investigated, and the type of hypothesis being tested.[1]

Of course, practically speaking, there will also be other important considerations to keep in mind, such as the availability of data, time constraints, the cost, the feasibility of the study, and others that will also play an important role in determining the most appropriate design to implement. In any case, the choice of study design (i.e., the methodology) should always be justified by a strong scientific and clinical rationale.

In this section, we will present the three traditional observational studies:

1. the cohort study,
2. the case-control study,
3. the cross-sectional study.

Then, we will introduce more advanced study designs including:

1. the nested case-control study,
2. the case-cohort study,
3. a few variations of the self-controlled study.

The advantages and limitations of each of these designs will also be presented in the case reports provided below. Table 3.3 outlines various measures of risk that are commonly used in pharmacoepidemiologic research. These measures will be referenced throughout this section and therefore the table below can be used as a reference when required. For further information regarding the definition of each risk presented in Table 3.3, please consult Annex 2.

3.4.2.1 The Prospective Cohort Study

Prospective cohort study (PCS) is a powerful observational study and, when conducted correctly, carries the greatest strength in terms of level of evidence relative to the other observational study designs. The PCS is preplanned and designed according to the research question addressed (see Annex 2).

The first step is to identify a sample study population. Ideally the sample population should be representative of the target population to which conclusions will be generalized. This is particularly important when conducting a descriptive study, but when conducting an analytical study it is important to enroll patients that are most likely to develop the outcome to ensure an adequate number of patients developing the outcome. The sample population chosen is referred to as the cohort under investigation.

At the onset of the study, none of the participants should have the outcome of interest; however, all patients should be equally at risk of developing the outcome. Baseline data are collected on all subjects including exposure assessment. It documents other important covariates that could have an impact on developing the outcome such as age, gender, the use of concomitant medications, relevant medical history, and others. These measurements, as well as when and/or if the outcome occurs, are also documented throughout the study.

TABLE 3.3 Measures of Frequency and Risk Estimation Commonly Used in Pharmacoepidemiologic Studies[1,24–25]

Measure of Risk	Explanation	Formula
Prevalence • Point prevalence • Period prevalence	The total number of cases that exist in the study population at a specific time point (i.e., *the point prevalence*) or over a period of time (i.e., *period prevalence*). This measure is used to estimate the disease burden.	$\text{Prevalence} = \frac{\text{\# of cases}}{\text{N}}$
Incidence • Cumulative incidence (CI) • Incidence rate (IR)	The number of new cases that developed during the study period.	$\text{Incidence} = \text{\# of new cases}$ $\text{CI} = \frac{\text{Incidence}}{\text{\# of persons at risk}}$ $\text{IR} = \frac{\text{Incidence}}{\text{Person–Time}}$
Absolute risk difference (ARD) (also referred to as the attributable risk)	This is an absolute measure of risk that quantifies the difference in risk observed in the exposed group versus the unexposed group.	$\text{ARD} = \text{CI (E)} - \text{CI (UE)}$
Number needed to treat (NNT)/Number needed to harm (NNH)	Used to determine the number of people needed to be treated for one person to experience a positive effect (i.e., NNT) or for one person to experience a negative effect (i.e., NNH).	$\text{NNT or NNH} = \frac{1}{\text{ARD}}$

Continued

TABLE 3.3 Measures of Frequency and Risk Estimation Commonly Used in Pharmacoepidemiologic Studies[1,24–25]—cont'd

Measure of Risk	Explanation	Formula
Relative risk (RR)	Used to determine the risk in one group as compared to another; most commonly it gives the ratio in the risk of the exposed population versus the unexposed population.	$RR = \frac{CI(E)}{CI(UE)}$
Relative risk reduction (RRR)	Used to determine the relative difference in risk in the exposed group compared to the unexposed group.	$RRR = \frac{CI\ (E) - CI\ (UE)}{CI\ (UE)}$
Odds ratio (OR)	Used to determine the odds of experiencing the outcome in the exposed group compared to the odds of experiencing the same outcome in the unexposed group.	$OR = \frac{\frac{\#\ of\ cases\ (E)}{\#\ of\ cases\ (UE)}}{\frac{\#\ of\ noncases\ (E)}{\#\ of\ noncases\ (UE)}}$
Incidence rate ratio (IRR)	Similar to the RR. However it compared the incident rate instead of cumulative incidence and therefore includes a consideration of person-time.	$IRR = \frac{IR\ (E)}{IR\ (UE)}$

E, exposed; *UE*, unexposed.

3.4.2.2 The Retrospective Cohort Study

A retrospective cohort study (RCS) uses the same methodology. However, the study is not preplanned and instead of following subjects forward into the future, they are followed backward into the past. To do this, an investigator goes back in time to identify a preexisting cohort that had been followed in the past for another purpose (see Annex 2).

Historical records of the entire cohort are examined to identify which subjects were exposed or not at the onset of the study and which of these subjects reported having the outcome at the end of the follow-up (see Annex 2).

Alternatively, if additional follow-up is required, the investigators could choose to continue to follow the patients identified in the cohort in the future. In this case, the cohort design would be a combination of both retrospective and prospective components. The RCS is not as methodologically strong as the PCS for one reason: the RCS is not preplanned study; therefore, the historical records may not have been structured to capture exposure and outcome details to the same level of accuracy. Also, the historical records may not have collected data on important covariates; therefore, when conducting any analysis it would not be possible to adjust for these potential confounders, which may distort the obtained measures of association.

RCS is advantageous over the PCS for practical reasons: the RCS must be cheaper and less resource intensive than the PCS and the analysis of data can be carried out immediately (in a PCS the investigator must allow sufficient time to elapse so that the outcome can occur). The cohort study, whether prospective or retrospective, is considered among the strongest observational designs because it allows the investigator to establish a clear temporal sequence where the exposure precedes the outcome. This is a crucial component for establishing causality.

Fig. 3.1 below shows a schematic representation of the PCS design. When conducted retrospectively, the diagram does not change. However, the investigators began their analysis after the patients have already developed the outcome (right side of diagram) and worked their way backward to assess which subjects were exposed versus unexposed.

3.4.2.2.1 The Measure of Risk in Cohort Studies

If the purpose of the study is descriptive, measures such as the **cumulative incidence** or **incidence rate** will be calculated to describe the frequency of the outcome occurrence. **Cumulative incidence** is a proportion that is calculated by dividing the number of new cases that developed by the total number of people at risk. This is a typical measurement when the cohort being followed is fixed (see Annex 2).

However, cumulative incidence is not always the best descriptive measure to use. First, when following patients over time, several patients may become

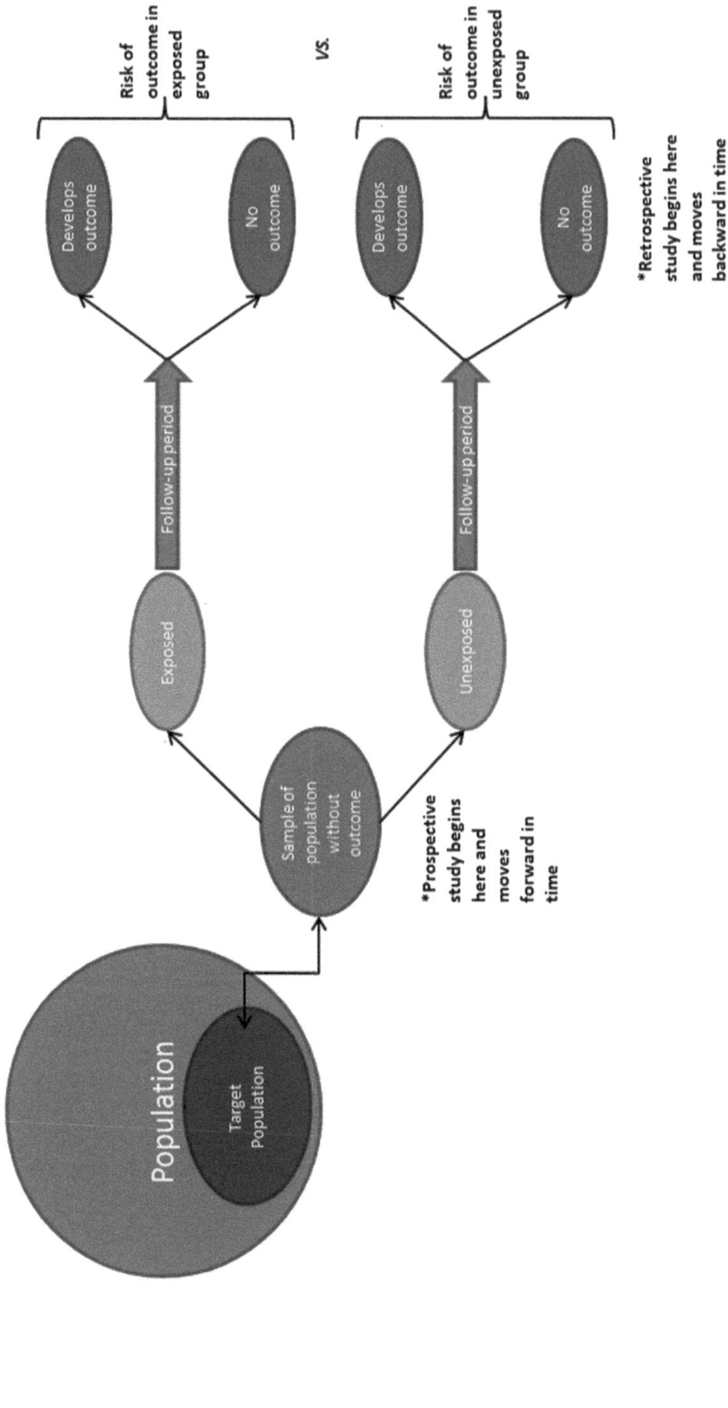

FIGURE 3.1 Schematic representation of a traditional cohort study design.

lost to follow-up (either because they drop out or due to death) and the calculation of the cumulative incidence becomes distorted. Second, when the cohort is dynamic, which means that a person can enter and leave the study at various time points, the time each person contributes to the study must be accounted for. In these situations, it is more informative to calculate the **incident rate** (see Annex 2).

The incidence rate differs from the cumulative incidence because it includes a time component, which accounts for how long each person contributed to the study. This measure is called person-time and is commonly reported as person-years, which refers to the number of years the subject was followed during the study and each person may contribute a different value of person-time (see Annex 2).

To calculate the incident rate, the number of cases is divided by the sum of total patient-time contributed by all subjects followed in the study. The nature of the cohort study and the research question submitted will determine which of the two measures is best to use.

When the purpose of the cohort study is analytical, the cohort is divided into two groups based on their exposure status. The occurrence of developing the outcome in the exposed group can be compared with the occurrence in the unexposed group.

When cumulative incidence between both groups is compared, the resulting measure of association is called the **relative risk (RR)**, whereas when the incidence rate is compared, the resulting measure of association is called the **incidence rate ratio (IRR)** (see Annex 2).

Statistical tests can be used to determine whether the difference between groups (i.e., the RR/IRR) is statistically significant. The above measures are relative; however, absolute measures can also be calculated and are crucial for conveying clinically relevant information.

The **absolute risk difference (ARD)** (also called **attributable risk)** is a measure used to show the difference in the cumulative incidence between the exposed and unexposed group. The reciprocal of the ARD gives us a measure called the **number needed to treat (NNT)** or the **number needed to harm (NNH)**. Both the NNT and NNH are calculated the same way but are used for different scenarios. Again, Chapter 4 below would be very helpful to help the readers understand these important concepts.

When, for example, a study is conducted to investigate the association between a harmful adverse event such as myocardial infarction and exposure to drug X, the reciprocal of the ARD (i.e., 1/ARD) will yield the NNH, which can be interpreted as the number of patients that need to be exposed to drug X for one patient to experience myocardial infarction.

A higher value of NNH implies better safety. On the other hand, if a study is conducted to investigate the effectiveness of drug X in preventing stroke, the reciprocal of the ARD will yield the NNT, which can be interpreted as the number of patients that need to be exposed to drug X for one patient to benefit.

TABLE 3.4 Contingency Table, Drug Z, and Aplastic Anemia

	Aplastic Anemia (i.e., Outcome Present)	No Aplastic Anemia (i.e., Outcome absent)
Exposed to drug Z	a = 23	b = 156
Not exposed to drug Z	c = 54	d = 640

Consider the following hypothetical data obtained from a cohort study designed to assess the association between drug Z and aplastic anemia (Table 3.4):

In this example, the RR compares the ratio of the risk of aplastic anemia among the exposed group to that among the unexposed group. The calculation is shown below:

$$\begin{aligned}\text{Relative Risk (RR)} &= (a/a+b)/(c/c+d) \\ &= (23/23+156)/(54/54+640) \\ &= 0.128/0.079 \\ &= 1.62\end{aligned}$$

Based on this calculation, we can conclude that exposure to drug Z results in a 62% increase in aplastic anemia. A 95% confidence interval or another statistical test should always be performed to determine whether the observed association is statistically significant. This is true for all subsequent calculations as well.

Absolute measures of risk can also be useful. In a cohort study the attributable risk (AR) (also called ARD) can be calculated by measuring the difference in the risk of aplastic anemia in the exposed group and that in the unexposed group. See the calculation below:

$$\begin{aligned}\text{Attributable Risk (AR)} &= (a/a+b) - (c/c+d) \\ &= 0.128 - 0.079 \\ &= 0{:}\ 05\end{aligned}$$

Based on this result we can conclude that the risk of developing aplastic anemia in the exposed group was 5% higher than in the unexposed group. The ARDs are often important for clinical interpretation of the results and should be considered in combination with the RR.

In determining the attributable risk, you can calculate the NNT/NNH. When the ARD is positive, it means the risk is higher in the exposed group. The NNT/NNH tells us how many patients need to be exposed to produce one adverse event of the outcome that should be investigated. Alternatively, if the ARD is negative, which means the risk of the outcome is lower in the exposed group, the NNT/NNH tells us how many patients need to be treated to prevent one adverse event of aplastic anemia. The NNT can be calculated as shown below:

$$\text{Number needed to treat (NNT)} = 1/\text{Attributable Risk}$$
$$= 1/0{:}\ 05$$
$$= 20$$

The NNT is a very valuable tool for the clinical interpretation of results obtained from a cohort study. In this case an NNT of 20 implies that 20 patients need to be exposed to drug Z for one event of aplastic anemia to occur. If drug Z is only exposed to very few patients, it may not be a cause for concern, but more likely drug Z will be used by a large number of people, in which case of aplastic anemia may present as a significant health concern.

3.4.2.3 The Case-Control Study

The case-control study uses a retrospective design to compare exposure history between two groups: one with the outcome of interest and the other without the outcome. This is different from the cohort study, which compares outcome status between two groups that differ in terms of exposure (see Annex 2).

Cases (i.e., patients with the outcome) are identified first and then for each case, a control (i.e., patient without the outcome) is identified. The control should be as similar to the case as possible, with only one main difference: the outcome status. The study can be done using a technique called matching. A 1:1 case-control ratio is described here. However, many studies will identify more than one control per case.

Once the cases and controls have been identified, the exposure status prior to the date of onset of the outcome in the case is assessed for both the case and matched control.

To illustrate this concept, consider the following example, Robinson et al.[26] wanted to investigate the association between exposure to the 5 α-reductase inhibitors and the risk of prostate cancer in Swedish men. In this study, cases (i.e., Swedish men with prostate cancer) were identified from the National Prostate Cancer Registry and for each case of prostate cancer, five matched controls (i.e., Swedish men without prostate cancer) were identified from the background population.

Previous exposure to the 5 α-reductase inhibitors for all cases and controls were assessed by extracting data from the Swedish Prescribed Drug Registry.

Fig. 3.2 below shows a schematic representation of the case-control study.

Typically case-control studies, as in the case of the example above, quantify the association between the exposure and outcome by comparing the odds of being exposed among the cases with the those among the controls. This risk measure is called the **odds ratio (OR)**. If we are investigating the

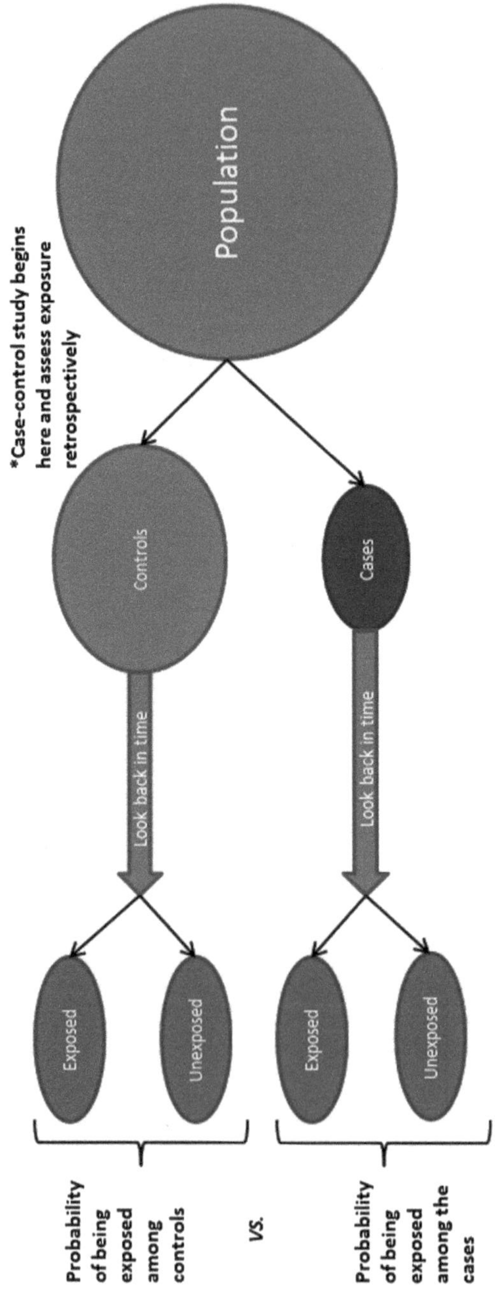

FIGURE 3.2 A schematic representation of a typical case-control study.

TABLE 3.5 Contingency Table, Drug A, and Outcome X

	Cases (i.e., Has Outcome X)	Controls (i.e., Does Not Have Outcome X)
Exposed to drug A	a = 20	b = 35
Not exposed to drug A	c = 100	d = 300

association between exposure to drug A and outcome X in a case-control study, the following results are obtained (Table 3.5):

Statistical analysis of the results obtained from the study is performed to quantify the association between the exposure and outcome. The odds of being exposed among the cases are compared to those among the controls. This risk measure is referred to as the OR as shown in the calculation below:

$$\begin{aligned}\text{Odds Ratio (OR)} &= (a/c)/(b/d) = a * d/b * c \\ &= (20 * 300)/(35 * 100) \\ &= 1.71\end{aligned}$$

Notice that the incidence, prevalence, RR, IRR, and ARD cannot be calculated in a case-control study. The population sample of the study is based on the identification of cases, which means the study sample is not representative of the entire population at risk.

Thus there are no data on the denominator that would be required for the above measures to be calculated. Case-control studies are clearly more limited than the cohort study because many important measures of risk/association cannot be calculated. However, when the outcome is very rare, the OR closely approximates the RR. Also, the interpretation of an OR is less intuitive than the RR.

A case-control study is more prone to biases than the cohort study. First of all, recall bias can distort the results. This occurs when the cases and controls are asked retrospectively about their exposure and provide inaccurate responses that are a form of information bias (see Annex 2). This type of bias is only an issue if the cases and controls differ in their ability to accurately report exposure. Selection bias can also be a problem if the cases and controls are not comparable.

To solve this type of bias, matching techniques are used when every case enrolled in the study is matched with one more control that is similar to the case in terms of various characteristics. Despite its limitations, the case control is an excellent design to use when the outcome investigated is rare because it is less costly than a cohort study and the results can be obtained far more quickly.

3.4.2.4 The Cross-Sectional Study

The cross-sectional study is an observational study that assesses exposure and the outcome at one specific point in time in a sample population. There is no prospective or retrospective follow-up. Both the RR and the OR can be calculated to describe the association between the exposure and the outcome. The incidence and prevalence, important descriptive measures, can also be calculated from a cross-sectional study.

The cross-sectional study cannot be used to infer causality because a temporal sequence cannot be established. Nevertheless, this type of study is used to generate descriptive statistics regarding the disease/outcome burden in a population, or to determine background exposure rates. All of which can be very useful, especially during the premarket phase of a product's life cycle. Fig. 3.3 below shows a schematic representation of a cross-sectional study.

3.5 ADVANCED OBSERVATIONAL STUDY DESIGNS

3.5.1 Nested Case-Control Studies[27,28]

As the name suggests, a nested case-control study is a hybrid of the cohort and case-control studies, whereas a case-control study is conducted within a pre-existing cohort. In this type of study, all the cases occurring in a cohort are identified. Controls (i.e., those who did not yet develop the outcome) are then selected (see Annex 2).

Each case is matched to one or more controls, generally four or five controls are selected for every case identified. Whether it is chosen according to age, data of entry into cohorts, the length of time in the cohort, etc., the type of matching is an essential component of the nested case-control study as it serves to minimize confounding at the design stage. It should also be noted that a selected control could also become a case later on as a follow-up continues and that one subject may be chosen as a control for more than one case.

A nested case-control is advantageous essentially because it minimizes the problems associated with a case-control study by adopting the characteristics of a cohort study. Yet, it can be conducted with limited resources and is both time and cost-efficient.

Because the source population of the cases and controls is the same in a nested case-control study (which is usually not the case in a typical case-control study), selection bias is reduced. Recall bias is also reduced because the data would have been collected prospectively, instead of having cases recall of their exposure, thus reducing errors regarding the misclassification of exposure status.

The disadvantage of the nested case-control study lies in the fact that the cohort was not designed to answer the question investigated by the nested

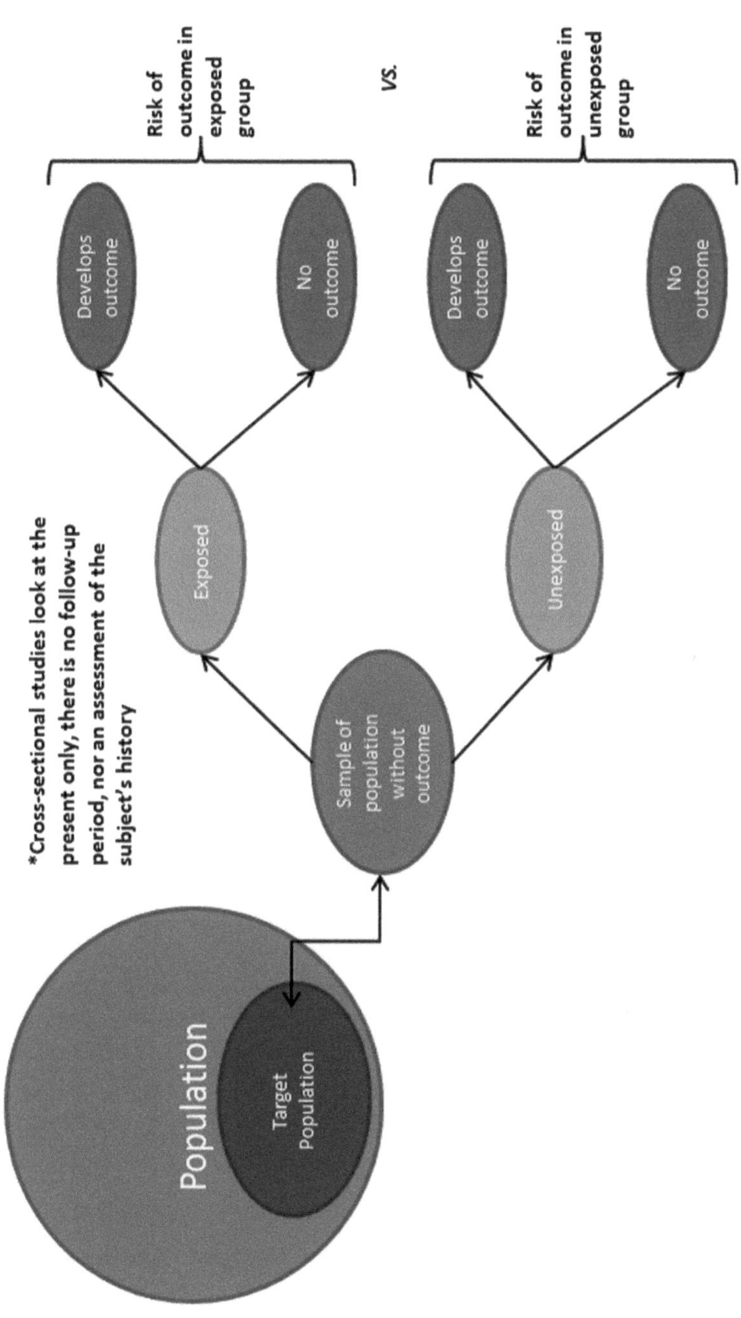

FIGURE 3.3 A schematic representation of a cross-sectional study.

case-control study, so important data regarding risk factors (relevant covariates) may not have been recorded adequately.

In this situation, it would be impossible to correct and adjust the potential confounding variables. In this regard, the nested case-control study is methodologically weaker than the traditional PCS.

Consequently, if important covariance data are collected appropriately, this type of study design has a major advantage over the traditional cohort study in that it can provide methodologically strong findings in a faster and less resource-intensive way.

In this type of study design the **OR** is used to quantify the measure of association. To obtain a better understanding on how this type of design is used for pharmacoepidemiologic research, the reader is invited to consult the methodology section of the current studies that have been performed using this design (see Annex 2).

Some examples include the Boursi et al.[29] (2014) study describing the association between exposure to digoxin and the increased risk of colorectal cancer and the study from Ishiguro et al.[30] (2014) investigating the relationship between antipsychotic drug use and the risk of venous thromboembolism. Both articles have been published in the Pharmacoepidemiologic Drug Safety Journal, which includes many other examples of the application of the nested case-control study. Other examples illustrating this concept are provided below in Chapter 4.

3.5.2 Case-Cohort Studies[28]

Similar to the nested case-control study, a case-cohort study is also a hybrid design taking elements of both the case-control and cohort studies. Similar to the case-control study, in the case-cohort, all cases in a specific cohort are identified at first and their exposure is assessed. Then out of the entire cohort enrolled at the beginning of the study, a random sample is obtained and exposure status is determined so that the distribution of exposure is the same as the distribution in the entire cohort (see Annex 2).

The advantage is that by taking only a random sample, it is more time efficient and less resource intensive to obtain exposure status on a significantly smaller segment of the entire cohort. **Incidence** and **RR** can thus be calculated. Case-cohort studies are far less common than the other designs for pharmacoepidemiologic research. However, it is nonetheless important to be familiar with the design.

3.5.3 Self-Control Studies

There are a few variations of the self-controlled observational study design that are commonly used for pharmacoepidemiologic research. Hallas and Pottegard[31] provide an excellent summary in their article published in the Journal of Internal Medicine.

This section will present the principles behind self-controlled studies in general and then discuss two specific examples: the case-crossover design and the self-controlled case series design.

The main weakness of observational studies used for pharmacoepidemiologic research is that comparisons are being made between subjects who have and who have not been exposed to a specific drug. However, because drugs are not randomly assigned to subjects as in the case of RCTs, it is more likely that subjects exposed to a drug differ in significant ways from subjects who have not been exposed to the drug.

Despite the various methods and precautions that can be taken to account for these differences between the groups, there is always a risk that the associations observed between an exposure and a risk are caused by some unaccounted difference between the two groups as opposed to the exposure to the drug itself.

This is true for virtually all the designs discussed above. To address this specific issue, the observational self-controlled studies have been proposed as they are especially useful when assessing drug exposure.

The self-controlled observational studies do not compare between two different groups of people but instead compares the time each individual subject was exposed to the drug as compared to the time when the individual was not exposed to the drug. Therefore each subject acts as his/her own control.

In a case-crossover design, each subject is his or her own control. As such, exposure is assessed during the period when the subject experienced the event. Then exposure is also assessed at a reference point in time when the subject did not experience the event. If a subject was not exposed either to the time of the event or the reference point, he is removed from the study analysis.

Similarly, if the subject was exposed to both the time of the event and during the reference period, he is also excluded. The remaining sample is compared and an OR can be expressed in terms of calculating the ratio of those exposed only during the time of the outcome and those exposed only during the reference period.

The self-controlled case series design is best understood as a variant of the traditional cohort study. In a self-controlled case series design, the case acts as its own control; however, instead of assessing exposure history at predefined reference dates, the subject's entire exposure history throughout a specific period is assessed. This also includes exposure ascertainment even after the event has resolved.

As such, instead of the unidirectional nature of the case-crossover study, this design adopts a bidirectional approach. In this type of study the **IRR** can be calculated. To obtain a better understanding of these designs and other variants of the self-controlled study consult the study by Hallas and Pottegard,[31] which provides a comprehensive overview of the self-controlled designs used for pharmacoepidemiologic research including a discussion on the strengths and weaknesses of each.

3.6 BIAS AND CONFOUNDING FACTORS

In the previous section we outlined various study designs that can be used to carry out pharmacoepidemiologic research. While the description of each study is fairly straightforward, there is a variety of errors that can occur at almost every stage of the proposed studies (i.e., during the conception, design, data collection, analysis, interpretation, reporting, the review of data, and even the publication) (see Annex 2 and Chapter 4).

When these errors cause the estimated measure of risk to systematically deviate from the true value of the measure, the study and its findings are considered biased.[6] When the deviation biases the results *toward the null hypothesis*, the measure is considered an underestimate, and when the deviation biases the results *away from the null hypothesis*, the measure is considered an overestimate.

Similarly, confounding occurs when an observed association between an exposure and outcome is due to a third factor that is responsible for causing the exposure and the outcome. Thus when this third factor is not accounted for, an association between the exposure and outcome is observed, although they are not truly associated with one another.[32] The issue of bias and confounding can occur in both RCTs and observational studies.

However, because RCTs are highly controlled, many of the biases and confounding factors can be handled and controlled appropriately. Because epidemiology designs are traditionally observational with no intervention, the issue of bias and confounding is a greater methodological challenge. Also due to the inappropriate handling of these errors, the findings from pharmacoepidemiologic studies are often questioned and/or criticized.

Although many types of bias exist, three broad categories of bias will be briefly presented in the following section: selection bias, information/misclassification bias, and confounding. Most other types of biases form subgroups that go under one of these categories. The presentation of these examples will focus on specific types of bias that are especially troublesome when conducting pharmacoepidemiologic research. To get a better understanding of the impact of bias and confounding, please consult the case report # 6 in Chapter 4 and also Annex 2.

3.6.1 Selection Bias

Selection bias occurs when the study population is not representative of the target population so that the measure of risks/benefits does not accurately represent the target population to which conclusions are being extended.

Selection bias could occur because of an error in the procedure used to select subjects or if there are other reasons that could explain why some participants would want to participate in the study and not others, or if some participants are more likely to be selected than others (see Annex 2).

Selection bias occurs early on in epidemiology study during the recruitment of participants and subsequently in the process of retaining the participants for the duration of the study. Once selection bias occurs not much can be done, but sensitivity analyses can be performed.

To correct the bias, as such, it is especially important to ensure that selection bias is avoided when recruiting and retaining the sample population. Common examples of selection bias that occur in pharmacoepidemiologic research include: referral bias, self-selection bias, prevalence bias, and protopathic bias.[33–36]

Referral bias can occur in pharmacoepidemiologic research when, for example a patient is more likely to be recruited into a study due to his exposure status than a control patient with the same drug exposure status.[33–36]

Self-selection bias occurs when patients volunteer to enroll in a study because it is likely that their motivation for enrolling into the study makes them significantly different from the target population. Alternatively, self-selection bias could occur when patients decide to drop out of a study for specific reasons, as opposed to randomly. This is why loss to follow up in a cohort study is a crucial aspect in determining the validity of that study.[33–36]

Prevalence bias is introduced in a study when prevalent cases as opposed to incident cases are recruited into the study sample so that a distortion in the findings can arise because the association could be the result of the duration of the disease as opposed to the incident outcome itself.[33–36] One way to avoid this type of bias is to restrict the sample to incident cases only.

Finally, **protopathic bias** arises when the issue of reverse causality comes into question. This can occur, for example, when a drug is prescribed due to a headache while the headache itself was one of the early symptoms of some form of cancer. The study would show an association between the drug and the cancer, even though the first symptom (headache) occurred before exposure to the drug.[33–36]

3.6.2 Misclassification (Information) Bias

Misclassification bias refers to measurement errors made in classifying a subject's exposure status or outcome status. Misclassification bias can also occur when inaccuracies are made in collecting information on important covariates. The misclassification bias is considered nondifferential (random) when the chance of misclassification is equal to exposure or outcome status.

Typically **nondifferential bias** will bias the findings toward the null and thus produce a more conservative estimate, but this is not always the case: in some situations nondifferential bias can also bias the findings away from the null.

Differential misclassification bias (nonrandom) is even more troublesome and occurs when the probability of misclassification is higher in one group compared to the other. Differential misclassification bias is commonly referred to as **information bias**.

Information bias is common in pharmacoepidemiologic studies that use administrative claims or hospital discharge databases because the diagnostic codes used to classify exposure and outcomes are very limited and often contain inaccuracies. These types of errors can severely distort the findings. In such cases, electronic medical record databases are more useful because they contain significantly more details and are more accurate.

Recall bias, a type of information bias, is also common in case-control studies. Recall bias occurs when one group, likely the exposed, is more able to accurately recall its exposure than the control group that could have paid less attention to its previous exposure, but the reverse situation could also occur, particularly if stigma is associated with previous exposure.[33–36]

One type of especially common information bias found in pharmacoepidemiologic research that relies on administrative databases has been associated to the choice of exposure risk.[37,38]

When using administrative data it is often unclear to determine how long the patient took the drug and when he took the drug. To correct this, time-windows have to be established to reflect the number of days the subject could have been at an excess risk due to the prescribed health product. If the choice of the exposure risk window is too small or too long, misclassification will occur, thereby distorting the results.

Another example of a bias that occurs in pharmacoepidemiologic research is the **immortal time bias** occurring when a patient is considered exposed even though it is not plausible for him to have experienced the outcome yet.[39] For example, if in a cohort that is being followed over time and grouped into exposed and unexposed subgroups, an IRR is compared between both groups, but if many of the exposed patients only became exposed halfway through the study, then their time prior to exposure would inaccurately be classified as exposed time. When this type of mistake occurs, a misclassification of exposure status distorts the overall findings.

Suissa[39] has explored this issue in detail, and his article should be consulted for additional information on the immortal time bias. Additionally, the ENCePP's Guidelines on Methodological Standards in Pharmacoepidemiology also provide important information on various biases that can affect pharmacoepidemiologic study designs (see http://www.encepp.eu/standards_and_guidances). The discussion on biases presented in this section is not comprehensive, but the intention was to give an understanding of how errors can occur at various points in the execution of studies.

3.6.3 Confounding Factors

As mentioned previously, confounding occurs when an extraneous factor is responsible for a relationship observed between exposure and outcome. This can occur in a variety of ways and is especially problematic in observational study designs (see Annex 2).

If the two groups being compared differ in a specific way that is unaccounted for, an erroneous association can be observed. For example, consider a study that attempts to show that taking drug X increases your risk of developing lung cancer; the conclusions of the study suggest that drug X is indeed associated with an increased risk of lung cancer. In this case, the study is redone; however, important covariance information is recorded for all subjects including their smoking status.

Then, it becomes clear that 90% of the patients exposed to drug X were long-term smokers, whereas only 2% of patients were not exposed to drug X. When accounting for smoking status, the relationship between drug X and lung cancer no longer exist and in this situation smoking status was the confounder. This, of course, is an exaggerated example, but it shows that, if relevant information on important covariates is not recorded and unaccounted for, erroneous conclusions can be produced.

When conducting a retrospective case-control study, or when using large administrative databases with little data on covariates, sometimes it is impossible to adequately address the issue of confounding, which presents a major challenge in pharmacoepidemiologic research. Even when all information of relevant covariates is recorded and accounted for during data analysis, it is always possible that some unknown and therefore unrecorded factor could be responsible for the observed association. This is known as **residual confounding**.[33–36]

Confounding by indication is a particular challenge that often arises in pharmacoepidemiologic studies. This occurs when subjects are assigned to one treatment over another due to certain factors, prognosis, or severity of disease, as opposed to another treatment. When this occurs the cases and controls being compared in the study are inherently different from one group being at an increased risk before the event is exposed. This, of course, results in a distortion of the overall calculated measure of association. Several publications discuss this issue further and should be consulted to obtain a better understanding of this concept.[32]

Potential factors influencing the decision to prescribe—thus potentially leading to confounding-by-indication—may vary by physician and over time and involve a mix of clinical, functional, and behavioral patient characteristics.

The channeling of drug prescribing to certain patients may also occur as a result of guidelines or reimbursement restrictions favoring certain drugs.

While randomization balances the groups with respect to both known and unknown covariates, observational studies are limited with respect to the latter, making confounding an important issue. The development of new techniques, such as propensity scores and other matching algorithms, has enabled studies handling large numbers of potential confounders. In theory, many confounding factors unknown today could be identified with the discovery of the human genome, taken into account, and adjusted for.

Effect modification is another important concept that should be understood along with the ability to clearly distinguish between a confounder and an effect modifier. As its name suggests, an effect modifier refers to a third variable that modifies the relationship between exposure and outcome.

Kamangar[40] provides the following example regarding the drug abacavir (used to treat HIV-infected patients), as it turns out that exposure to this drug is associated with increased severe/fatal hypersensitivity, but this association is only seen in patients with a certain genetic allele. Thus, the conclusion is that the effect of abacavir is modified by the presence of certain genetic alleles. Kamangar's article on Effect Modification in Epidemiology and Medicine is an excellent resource for those interested in understanding more about effect modification.

3.7 CRITICAL APPRAISAL IN PHARMACOEPIDEMIOLOGIC RESEARCH

When introducing the various study designs that can be used for pharmacoepidemiologic research, we stated that the appropriate choice of study design is critical. However, this alone is not sufficient to produce good-quality research. Even after choosing an appropriate study design, the study must also be conducted correctly because as we showed in the previous section, the issue of bias and confounding is a main source of criticism against epidemiologic research.

There are many critical appraisal tools and checklists that can be used to assess the quality of a study. A good example is STROBE (**S**trengthening **t**he **r**eporting of **ob**servational studies in **E**pidemiology), which can be accessed at the following link: http://www.strobe-statement.org/index.php?id=available-checklists.

Because critical appraisal tools already exist and are easily accessible. In the next section, instead of presenting an exhaustive list, only some of the most important considerations that should be taken into account before accepting the findings produced from a pharmacoepidemiologic study are discussed.

The goal of pharmacoepidemiologic studies, broadly speaking, is to quantify an association between exposure to a therapeutic product and either a beneficial effect or a negative consequence, such as one or more adverse events. Thus, when critically appraising a pharmacoepidemiologic study, we ultimately want to assess both the validity and the accuracy of the quantified measures produced from the study. There are two types of validity to consider: the first is internal validity and the secondly is external validity.

Internal validity essentially describes how well the study was performed and therefore how valid the conclusion from the study is. Internal validity is compromised when bias and confounders are not handled correctly, and thus the measures of association are distorted away from the true values.

The way the sample was recruited into the study and the number that was retained is extremely important for establishing internal validity. Additionally, the choice of comparators in a pharmacoepidemiologic study is another critical component.

Because pharmacoepidemiologic deals with drug use in the real world, it is likely that those cases exposed to the drug are significantly different from patients who have not been exposed to the drug. These differences must be accounted for in the analysis to ensure that the conclusions from the study are indeed valid.

Protocols taken to minimize information bias are equally important because misclassification can have a major impact on the validity of a study. The exposure and outcome should be clearly defined and if proxy end points are being used, it is important that they are validated.

The way in which subjects exposure and outcome status is ascertained should be clearly outlined and consideration should be placed on whether the methods used did not introduce any misclassification bias into the study.

External validity, on the other hand, refers to how generalizable the findings are to a larger, broader, target population. External validity is thus dependent on how representative the sample population is to the external study. In an RCT, for example, internal validity is very high, but external validity is low.

Observational studies often have better external validity, but are not as internally valid because they are not highly controlled. Accuracy or precision of the measurement is also an important consideration. If a study includes an insufficient sample size, the generated measure of association will have a wide confidence interval and therefore will not be extremely useful. Thus, another important consideration when appraising a pharmacoepidemiologic study is the number of subjects enrolled in the study and whether the sample size was sufficient.

However the data analysis strategy used must be carefully analyzed. As the saying goes, if data are tortured for long enough, eventually you can make the data say whatever you want. Thus, it is important that the data analysis strategy along with clear hypotheses is made a priori to the conduct of the study to avoid data torturing.

Other considerations, such as how missing data and losses to follow up were handled can also have major impacts to the overall findings in a pharmacoepidemiologic study. Of course, in this section, only some important aspects to consider when critically appraising an epidemiologic study were very briefly covered. As mentioned, there are several tools and preexisting checklists that provide a systematic and step-by-step approach to critically appraise the findings from clinical research, such as the STROBE Guidelines, which can be accessed at the following link: http://www.strobe-statement.org/index.php?id=available-checklists.

3.8 SOURCES OF DATA FOR PHARMACOEPIDEMIOLOGIC RESEARCH

Data collected for epidemiologic studies can be obtained either through primary or secondary means. Primary data collection refers to collecting data specifically for the purposes of the study, whereas secondary data collection uses data that have already been collected for a different purpose.[37]

Today, due to technological advancements and the creation of databases, secondary data sources are more commonly used for pharmacoepidemiologic research. This is mainly due to logistical reasons (i.e., less costly and more time efficient) and also because of certain benefits for the validity of the study especially when the use of very large sample sizes is necessary.[41]

Common sources of secondary data used for pharmacoepidemiologic are administrative claim databases (insurance claims, medical claims, and drug-dispensing pharmacy data) and medical record databases (electronic health records). Strom, Kimmel, and Hennessy's textbook *Pharmacoepidemiology* (5th ed.) contains an in-depth review of these secondary data sources, including a discussion on strengths and limitations of each.

For additional details, consult the *FDA Guidance for Industry: Best Practices for Conducting and Reporting Pharmacoepidemiology Safety Studies using Electronic Health care Data* (http://www.fda.gov/downloads/Drugs/GuidanceComplianceRegulatoryInformation/Guidances/UCM243537.pdf). Work by Schneeweiss and Avorn can also be reviewed for a better understanding of the limitations associated with using secondary data sources for pharmacoepidemiologic research.[42]

Although secondary data sources are indeed advantageous in many ways, databases do not always contain sufficient data required to adequately answer a specific research question.

Primary data collection is particularly advantageous because all data collection is tailored toward the specific research question, thus, allowing a more accurate assessment of outcome and exposure data. Primary data collection is also advantageous for the collection of relevant confounding factors that are often not captured in administrative databases. RCT and prospective cohort studies are two examples of study designs that typically require the collection of primary data.

Primary data collection has its limitations, as it is often a costly, resource-intensive, and time-consuming procedure. To render primary data collection more efficient especially in the context of pharmacoepidemiologic research, certain systems can be implemented to collect data on an ongoing basis as in case-control surveillance and patient registries, for example.

A case-control surveillance study uses a network of various sources to track cases of a particular condition on an ongoing, prospective basis. For example, a hospital-based case-control surveillance study conducted in Berlin included a network of 51 hospitals and was used to identify cases of idiopathic acute pancreatitis (IAP).

From this network, 102 cases of IAP were captured and compared with 750 controls. Because the case-control surveillance was prospective and ongoing, it was possible to further assess the identified cases using WHO-UMC causality assessment criteria and obtain details on drug exposure using face-to-face interviews.[43] These types of case-control surveillance networks are particularly useful for identifying and better characterizing safety signals. For more information regarding the use of case-control surveillance studies consult the work of Kaufman et al.[41]

Another example of ongoing data collection that can be used for pharmacoepidemiologic research is patient registries (discussed above). Registries usually enroll a large number of patients mainly based on a similar characteristic depending on the purpose of the registry.

For example, a regulatory agency may request a patient registry for all patients exposed to a newly approved health product to better characterize the safety and efficacy of the product.

Alternatively, a patient registry can be formed on the basis of disease status where, for example, patients with a specific type of cancer are enrolled.[37] The scope (inclusion/exclusion criteria) in a registry can vary depending on the purpose: some registries may collect data on 100% of the target population, whereas others may enroll patients on a voluntary basis.

Registries are made up of prospectively collected data obtained from clinical and medical data collected from health-care providers, from electronic or paper health-care records and/or administrative claims data. As time goes on, the data collected can be modified to reflect new or changing research questions. In any case, registries collect detailed clinical information on each patient and thus serve as a rich source of data that can be used to conduct cohorts and case-control studies.[44a]

3.9 EXPERIMENTAL STUDY DESIGNS

3.9.1 The Large Simple Trial

Of all experimental designs, the RCT is the gold standard study because of its ability to provide unbiased estimates benefits and risks associated with a health product. A detailed discussion on the conduct of an RCT (including the different types: double-blind, parallel, crossovers, etc.) is out of the scope of this chapter (see the ICH Guidance Document E6: Good Clinical Practice and E8: General Considerations for Clinical Trials for more information on clinical trials).

Two notable features of the RCT are the use of randomization and blinding. These techniques are used to minimize confounding and biases to produce accurate estimates (high internal validity). The health product treatment and comparator health product or placebo are randomly assigned to patients to create two comparable groups and blinding techniques are used so that the patient's response and the investigator's assessment are not affected by knowing whether the patient received the treatment drug or the comparator.

These types of studies often utilize complex designs that are resource intensive and costly. As such, these trials are mainly limited for use in the preapproval setting to show unbiased estimates of efficacy, which is required to grant marketing authorization for the product. However, RCTs can be adapted for use as phase IV postmarket drug safety studies, as in the case of the large simple trial (LST).

LSTs are RCTs that enroll a large number of patients using broad inclusion/exclusion criteria to allow for a heterogeneous population and is more reflective of use in the real-world setting. A large number of patients are required to provide enough power to the study and to adequately identify safety issues despite a heterogeneous population and also to allow the identification of rare adverse events or small changes in frequencies of commonly reported adverse events. Furthermore, the follow-up period for an LST can continue in the long term if the purpose of the study is to assess long-term safety.

An RCT designed to demonstrate clinical efficacy is costly, resource-intensive, and utilizes complex designs. Thus, it would simply not be feasible to conduct an equally complex RCT clinical trial in the postmarket setting, increase the length of the study, and increase the number of patients enrolled.

As such, the LST, as the name would suggest, utilizes a simple randomized design only. Primary end points are objective and easy to measure, data collection is kept to a minimum (only relevant and limited baseline and follow-up data are collected) and follow-up should be observational. This increases the feasibility of such a study and allows for an accurate and unbiased safety assessment.

The LST can be used to assess safety and/or effectiveness (keep in mind that effectiveness and efficacy are two different concepts). Van Ganse et al. (2005)[44b] published results from an LST to compare the tolerability of three OTC medications (acetaminophen, aspirin, and ibuprofen) using patient-reported adverse event data as the primary outcome in which 8677 patients were initially enrolled. The incidence of reported adverse events were calculated in each group and compared. The study concluded that this type of trial can provide sensitive information on adverse events and are especially useful for comparative safety assessments.

Given its methodological strengths, the LST is becoming an increasingly important component of phase IV postmarket safety research; however, the LST is not always an appropriate choice.

First, despite attempts to keep the LST simple to ensure feasibility, it remains a costly option and therefore is less attractive for sponsors to conduct, especially given that their product would have already received marketing authorization.

Second, the conduct of a clinical trial may be unethical in certain scenarios because you cannot administer an agent that knowingly causes harm to one group nor can one withhold a medication that would result in benefits to the patient. As such, for an LST to be acceptable, it has to meet the "uncertainty" criteria, which means that the administering physician must be unsure that the treatment option is best for the patient. Alternatively, others believe in the clinical equipoise criteria when the community of physicians is collectively unsure about which treatment option is best, not only for one individual patient but also for a group of patients as well.[45]

3.9.2 The N-Of-1 Trial

Real-world clinical practice differs from RCTs because health-care providers will experience unique challenges and/or unexpected outcomes when interacting with patients on an individual basis. As such, health-care providers often have to alter treatment strategies depending on the unique characteristics of their patient. RCTs may answer overall questions about clinical efficacy of a particular health product, but not necessarily about which health product will be the best for each specific patient and often with time, patients will not fit into the inclusion/exclusion criteria of a specific RCT.

Therefore the results may not be directly applicable. In such situations, health-care providers often end up conducting their own experiments on patients by trialing certain treatment options and adjusting therapy according to the patient's response.

To avoid misleading conclusions, a specific protocol has been developed to insure a methodologically sound conduct of these experimental trials on one individual. This type of trial is called the N-of-1 trial, which is essentially an RCT (most similar to the crossover design) performed on one individual patient.

Guyatt et al.[46] created a guide on how to conduct N-of-1 trials and should be referenced. To summarize: an N-of-1 trial is carried out on one patient to find the ideal treatment option for that patient. The comparison can be between an active drug and a placebo or a higher dose versus a lower dose of a medication. An N-of-1 trial may not always be appropriate, but when it is, the data obtained can be very useful in determining the effectiveness and safety of a therapy in a specific individual patient.[46]

3.10 SYSTEMATIC REVIEW AND METAANALYSIS

The systematic review and metaanalysis (SR/MA) are also important study designs used for pharmacoepidemiologic research. Although the SR/MA does not fall under the conventional understanding of a pharmacoepidemiologic observational study, they are an important tool that can be used for a variety of purposes to provide comprehensive evidence on a specific topic. These types of study designs will be further illustrated below on Chapter 4.

The systematic review differs from a traditional literature review in several ways. In a systematic review a very specific research question is asked at the onset of the study and then a wide set of databases and gray literature is systematically searched using specific search terms to identify relevant publications/articles according to a set of strict predefined inclusion/exclusion criteria. Once articles have been identified they undergo several other screening processes until a final set of articles are considered for the final analysis.

In a systematic review, the articles are not analyzed subjectively; data are instead extracted according to a premade template so that the data extracted from each study is consistent. These protocols eliminate the subjectivity of a normal traditional literature review and greatly increase the strength and reliability of the findings.

In some cases, when the studies included are very similar, the data from all the studies can be pulled together and reanalyzed: this is referred to as a metaanalysis. For more details on the conduct of SR/MA consult the Cochrane Handbook for Systematic Reviews of Interventions (http://community.cochrane.org/handbook).

Here are few examples of how the SR/MA can be beneficial for pharmacoepidemiologic research: if various studies explore the association between drug X and hepatotoxicity and if variability appears in the findings across the studies, then SR/MA can be used to determine why these inconsistencies exist.

Alternatively, if the research question being investigated concerns an adverse outcome that is uncommon or rare, SR/MA can gather all relevant studies and if applicable pool the results, it can be used to study the adverse outcome more efficiently.

Finally, another use of the SR/MA is to identify if subgroups exist in terms of treatment response or to identify the occurrence of adverse outcomes within the population being studied.[1] These are only a few examples that demonstrate the importance of the systematic review and metaanalysis.

3.10.1 The Grading System

When a systematic review has been well performed, we can establish some recommendations based on the grading of recommendations assessment, development, and evaluation (GRADE) system, i.e., the recommendations are graded according to the GRADE. GRADE offers two strengths of recommendation: strong and weak. The strength of recommendations is based on the quality of supporting evidence; degree of uncertainty about the balance between desirable and undesirable effects; degree of uncertainty or variability in values and preferences; and degree of uncertainty about whether the intervention represents a wise use of resources.

Strong recommendations are those for which the authors are confident that the desirable effects of an intervention outweigh its undesirable effects (strong recommendation for an intervention) or that the undesirable effects of an intervention outweigh its desirable effects (strong recommendation against an intervention). A strong recommendation implies that most individuals will be best served by the recommended course of action.

Weak recommendations are those for which the desirable effects probably outweigh the undesirable effects (weak recommendation for an intervention) or undesirable effects probably outweigh the desirable effects (weak recommendation against an intervention) but appreciable uncertainty exists. A weak recommendation implies that most people would want the recommended course of action but that many would not. For clinicians this means they must recognize that different choices will be appropriate for each individual, and they must help each person arrive at a management decision consistent with his/her values and preferences. Policy-making will require substantial debate and involvement of various stakeholders. Weak recommendations result when the balance between desirable and undesirable effects is small, the quality of evidence is lower, or there is more variability in the values and preferences of patients. Evidence is graded as high, moderate, low, or very low based on how likely further research is to change our confidence in the estimate of effect.

3.11 CONCLUSIONS

The designs used in pharmacoepidemiologic studies are not much different from those used in other areas of clinical epidemiology. However, because these studies are generally performed after a health product has been approved for marketing, pharmacoepidemiologic studies usually include substantially larger numbers of patients who are followed for a longer duration to add new useful active surveillance information.

A strong and useful pharmacoepidemiologic study is one that is designed in accordance to the question the researcher wants to answer. Unfortunately, there is no golden standard design that will perfectly fit with research questions; each pharmacoepidemiology study design has its strengths and advantages.

Over the years more and more data have become available in the constantly growing databases on prescription drugs. This has facilitated the development of pharmacoepidemiology, a dynamic research field that has undergone a more rapid development than many other research areas. There are several reasons why pharmacoepidemiology will remain recognized as one of the most dynamic and challenging research areas of clinical pharmacology. The data explosion in modern society will continue, and observational studies aimed at assessing the value of health products will be increasingly requested by payers, professionals, and patients. Future studies in pharmacoepidemiology must include specialist drugs used in the hospital setting and also be designed to address obstacles hindering the delivery of effective medicines to the patient. Pharmacoepidemiologic methods may also be valuable tools to address new challenges, such as the environmental impact of health products. A potential threat is that the increasing amounts of data available in registries may add fuel to the debate on confidentiality. On the other hand, strict application of privacy rules might hinder the further development of pharmacoepidemiology.

Ultimately, the choice of the study design is more a matter of maximizing the pros and minimizing the cons while considering limitations including the availability of data, the constraints of time, the cost, and the feasibility as well as several other important factors such as bias and confounding factors. In all cases, the choice of pharmacoepidemiologic design should always be supported by appropriate scientific or clinical justifications.

The availability of electronic health-care databases will enable researchers to identify a growing number of cases in which effectiveness does not match efficacy. This will challenge the actions of all concerned stakeholders including the industry, regulatory agencies, payers, and health-care providers. Risk management plans or risk evaluation and mitigation strategies are already required by EMA, the FDA, Health Canada, and other regulatory agencies as part of the medicine approval process to help ensure that the benefits of a particular medicine outweigh its risks. Observational studies will also be increasingly requested by reimbursement agencies and other payers to assess the value of health products. It is also likely that patients will demand better systems to monitor effectiveness and safety.

In the future, it is therefore likely that all new drugs will be monitored postmarketing. This monitoring may range from descriptive drug statistics to sophisticated comparative effectiveness studies, depending on the budget impact and level of uncertainty about the benefit–risk of the health product. The difficulties in conducting studies also indicate that the nature of the monitoring activities will be limited by the availability of data and competent pharmacoepidemiologists. Payers will also increasingly require health economic studies to assess the cost-effectiveness of the new premium-priced therapies compared to the existing standards. Increasing difficulties for national health services financing new expensive therapies such as cancer therapies will lead to the development of various risk-sharing models.

To conclude it is essential that the increasing amounts of data collected to monitor the utilization, effectiveness, and safety of new health products will be used to improve clinical decision-making.

The annex that follows defines most of the pharmacoepidemiologic terms mentioned in this chapter and provides a summary of the various topics that have been covered. Because pharmacoepidemiology works in synergy with pharmacovigilance for a better investigation of adverse drug reactions, some of the terms pertaining to pharmacovigilance have been included here. Most of the definitions provided below come from various ICH Guidelines and from some French and English publications, where needed.

REFERENCES

1. Strom B, Kimmel S, Hennessy Sean, eds. *Textbook of Pharmacoepidemiology*. 2nd ed. Sussex: John Wiley & Sons; 2013.
2. Canada Health. *Product Life Cycle*; December 12, 2011. From Health Canada: http://www.hc-sc.gc.ca/sr-sr/tech/biotech/health-prod-sante/prod_life-vie-eng.php.
3. Avorn J. In defense of pharmacoepidemiology – embracing the Yin and Yang of drug research. *N Engl J Med*. 2007;357:2219–2221.
4. Silverman SL. From randomized controlled trials to observational studies. *Am J Med*. 2009;122:114–120.
5. Ahmad SR. Adverse drug event monitoring at the Food and Drug Administration: your report can make a difference. *J Gen Intern Med*. 2003;18:57–60.
6. Porta M, ed. *A Dictionary of Epidemiology*. 5th ed. New York: Oxford University Press; 2008.
7. Rogers AS, Israel E, Smith CR. Physician knowledge, attitudes, and behaviour related to reporting adverse drug events. *Arch Intern Med*. 1988;148:1589–1592.
8. Scott HD, Rosenbaum SE, Water WJ, et al. Rhode Island physician's recognition and reporting of adverse drug reactions. *R I Med J*. 1987;70:311–316.
9. Belhekar MN, Santosh RT, Munshi RP. A study of agreement between the Naranjo algorithm and WHO-UMC criteria for causality assessment of adverse drug reactions. *Indian J Pharmacol*. 2014;46:117–120.
10. Doherty MJ. Algorithms for assessing the probability of an adverse drug reaction. *Respir Med CME*. 2009;2:63–67.
11. Montastruc JL, Sommet A, Bagheri H, Lapeyre-Mestre M. Benefits and strengths of the disproportionality analysis for identification of adverse drug reactions in a pharmacovigilance database. *Br J Clin Pharmacol*. 2011;72:905–908.
12. Bate A, Evans SJ. Quantitative signal detection using spontaneous ADR reporting. *Pharmacoepidemiol Drug Saf*. 2009;18:427–436.
13. Hauben M, Madigan D, Gerrits CM, Walsh L, Van Puijenbroek EP. The role of data mining in pharmacovigilance. *Expet Opin Drug Saf*. 2005;4:929–948.
14. Rothman KJ, Lanes S, Sacks ST. The reporting odds ratio and its advantages over the proportional reporting ratio. *Pharmacoepidemiol Drug Saf*. 2004;13:519–523.
15. Evans SJ, Waller PC, Davis S. Use of proportional reporting ratios (PRRs) for signal generation from spontaneous adverse drug reaction reports. *Pharmacoepidemiol Drug Saf*. 2001;10:483–486.

16. Bate A, Lindquist M, Edwards IR, et al. A Bayesian neural network method for adverse drug reaction signal generation. *Eur J Clin Pharmacol.* 1998;54:315–321.
17. Van Puijenbroek EP, Bate A, Leufkens HGM, Lindquist M, Orre R, Egberts AC. A comparison of measures of disproportionality for signal detection in spontaneous reporting systems for adverse drug reactions. *Pharmacoepidemiol Drug Saf.* 2002;11:3–10.
18. Szarfman A, Machado SG, O'Neill RT. Use of screening algorithms and computer systems to efficiently signal higher-than-expected combinations of drugs and events in the US FDA's spontaneous reports database. *Drug Saf.* 2002;25:381–392.
19. Bate A. Bayesian confidence propagation neural network. *Drug Saf.* 2007;7:623–625.
20. Szarfman A, Tonning JM, Doraiswamy PM. Pharmacovigilance in the 21st century: new systematic tools for an old problem. *Pharmacotherapy.* 2004;24:1099–1104.
21. Almenoff JS, DuMouchel W, Kindman A, Yang X, Fram D. Disproportionality analysis using empirical Bayes data mining: a tool for the evaluation of drug interactions in the post-marketing setting. *Pharmacoepiedmiol Drug Saf.* 2003;12:517–521.
22. Sakaeda T, Tamon A, Kadoyama K, Okuno Y. Data mining of the public version of the FDA adverse event reporting system. *Int J Med Sci.* 2013;10:796–803.
23. EMA. *Guidelines on the Use of Statistical Signal Detection Methods in the Eudravigilance Data Analysis System*; June 26, 2008. From European Medicines Agency: http://www.ema.europa.eu/docs/en_GB/document_library/Regulatory_and_procedural_guideline/2009/11/WC500011434.pdf.
24. Rothman KJ, Greenland S, Lash TL. In: Rothman KJ, ed. *Modern Epidemiology.* 3rd ed. Philadelphia, PA: Lippincott, Williams & Wilkins; 2008.
25. Quartey G, Wang J, Kim J. A review of risk measures in pharmacoepidemiology with tips for statisticians in the pharmaceutical industry. *Pharmaceut Stat.* 2011;10:548–553.
26. Robinson D, Garmo H, Bill-Axelson A, Mucci L, Holmberg L, Stattin P. Use of 5α-reductase inhibitors for lower urinary tract symptoms and risk of prostate cancer in Swedish men: nationwide, population based case-control study. *BMJ.* 2013;346:f3406.
27. Sedgwick P. Nested case-control studies: advantages and disadvantages. *BMJ.* 2014;348:g1532.
28. Ernster V. Nested case-control studies. *Prev Med.* 1994;23:587–590.
29. Boursi B, Haynes K, Mamtani R, Yang YX. Digoxin use and the risk of colorectal cancer. *Pharmacoepidemiol Drug Saf.* 2014;23(11):1147–1153. https://doi.org/10.1002/pds. 3717. Epub September 29, 2014.
30. Ishiguro C, Wang Z, Li L, Jick S. Antipsychoatic drugs and risk of idiopathic venous thromboembolism: a nested case-control study using the CPRD. *Pharmacoepidemiol Drug Saf.* 2014;23(11):1168–1175. https://doi.org/10.1002/pds. 3699. Epub September 7, 2014.
31. Hallas J, Pottegard A. Use of self-controlled designs in pharmacoepidemiology. *J Intern Med.* 2014;275:581–590.
32. Joseph K, Mehrabadi A, Lisonkova S. Confounding by indication and related concepts. *Curr Epidemiol Rep.* 2014;1:1–8.
33. Boccia S, La Torre G, Persiani R, D'Ugo D, van Duinj C, Ricciardi G. A critical appraisal of epidemiologic studies comes from basic knowledge: a reader's guide to assess potential for biases. *World J Emerg Surg.* 2007;2. https://doi.org/10.1186/1749-7922-2-7.
34. Delgado-Rodriguez M, Llorca J. Continuing professional Education: bias. *J Epidemiol Community Health.* 2004;58:635–641.
35. Csizmadi I, Collet JP, Boivin JF. Bias and confounding in pharmacoepidemiology. In: Strom B, ed. *Pharmacoepidemiology.* Sussex: Wiley; 2005:793–809.

36. Pannucci C, Wilkins E. Identifying and avoiding bias in research. *Plast Reconstr Surg.* 2010;126:619–625.
37. The European Network of Centres for Pharmacoepidemiology and Pharmacovigilance (ENCePP). Guide on Methodological Standards in Pharmacoepidemiology (Revision 3). EMA/95098/2010. Available at: http://www.encepp.eu/standards_and_guidances.
38. Van Staa T, Abenhaim L, Leufkens H. A study of the effects of exposure misclassification due to the time-window design in pharmacoepidemiologic studies. *J Clin Epidemiol.* 1994;47:183–189.
39. Suissa S. Immortal time bias in pharmacoepidemiology. *Am J Epidemiol.* 2008;167:492–499.
40. Kamanger F. Effect modification in epidemiology and medicine. *Arch Iran Med.* 2012;15:575–582.
41. Kaufman DW, Rosenberg L, Mitchell AA. Signal generation and clarification: use of case-control data. *Pharmacoepidemiol Drug Saf.* 2001;10:197–203.
42. Schneeweiss S, Avorn J. A review of uses of health care utilization databases for epidemiologic research on therapeutics. *J Clin Epidemiol.* 2005;58:323–337.
43. Douros A, Bronder E, Andersohn F, et al. Drug-induced acute pancreatitis: results from the hospital-based Berlin case-control surveillance study of 102 cases. *Aliment Pharmacol Ther.* 2013;7:825–834.
44a. Dreyer N, Velentgas P. Registries. In: Strom B, ed. *Pharmacoepidemiology.* Sussex: Wiley; 2012:331–346.
44b. Van Ganse E, Jones JK, Moore N, et al. A large simple clinical trial prototype for assessment of OTC drug effects using patient-reported data. *Pharmacoepidemiology and Drug Safety.* 2005;14:249–255.
45. Weijer C, Shapiro SH, Glass KC. Clinical equipoise and not the uncertainty principle is the moral underpinning of the randomised controlled trial. *BMJ.* 2000;321:756.
46. Guyatt G, Sackett D, Adachi J, et al. A clinician's guide for conducting randomized trials in individual patients. *CMAJ.* 1988;139:497–503.

Chapter 4

Case Studies

4.1 CASE REPORT # 1

4.1.1 The Concept of the Therapeutic Product Life Cycle Approach Applied to an Orphan Drug

Drug A is a monoclonal antibody with a high affinity against a genetically modified human interleukin and designed for the treatment of a rare genetic disorder or orphan disease. The sponsor has presented a new drug submission (NDS) to obtain authorization to market drug A for the treatment of this disease. As the head of the division in charge of reviewing this NDS, you want to be sure that a life cycle–based approach is in place for the evaluation of this submission (see Fig. 1.1 of chapter 1).

Question # 1: What are the main concepts related to the life cycle–based approach?

Among the following, which apply (yes)?

(A) Progressive knowledge about the product.
(B) Based on solid evidence.
(C) Good planning.
(D) Accountability (transparency).
(E) All of the above.

Answer: E.

The approach, based on the life cycle of the product (see Chapter 1, Fig. 1.1), aims to develop a framework that can facilitate access to new therapies through a continuous process of monitoring, evaluation, and dissemination of information on a health product especially concerning the benefits and risks associated with this product throughout its life cycle to ensure its optimal use and to maximize its benefits while minimizing its risks.

The first objective of this approach is to protect the public against the marketing of dangerous products and to encourage an optimal and safe use of health products in either in the development phase and/or following market authorization.[1,2]

(A) Progressive knowledge about the product. A life cycle–based approach is justified by the fact that knowledge about a product progresses with time. With this approach, rather than putting the regulatory priority on

Pharmacoepidemiology and Pharmacovigilance. https://doi.org/10.1016/B978-0-12-816183-8.00004-4

premarket assessment, a drug is evaluated throughout its life cycle with regard to its benefit/risk ratio, which includes both the pre- and postmarketing periods.[1,2]

(B) Based on solid evidence: The approach offers a decision-making process based on solid evidence. It requires not only data on efficacy and safety, but it also incorporates other kinds of evidence for a full assessment of the risks and benefits. This approach also provides flexibility to better inform those who must make a decision about the efficacy and safety of a health product and the pharmacovigilance of its adverse effects.[1,2]

(C) Good planning. It implies a well-structured strategic approach to generate and exchange add of continuous information throughout the life cycle of a health product. Among the potential benefits, it is essential to notice that this approach is intended, among other things, (1) to reduce of the length of time it takes to access the best possible health product for patients, (2) to acquire a systematic collection of useful data in the setting and monitoring of the benefit/risk ratio during the life cycle of the product, (3) to increase efficiency in the development of health products by industry, (4) to optimize the management of resources, and (5) to ensure better prevention of adverse effects of drugs and other activities.[1,2]

(D) Accountability (transparency) is defined as a permanent requirement to justify decisions made by regulatory agencies, including Health Canada, the Food and Drug Administration (FDA), the European Medicine Agency (EMA) and others, including the health products industry. The central idea is that over time, the level of knowledge increases about the risks and benefits of a drug; about its use by specific and unique populations, including children, pregnant and breastfeeding women, the elderly, and others; about its interaction with other drugs; and about its new indications.

As presented in Chapter 1, Fig. 1.1, this process recognizes the importance of accountability (transparency) and good communication, and close collaboration between all parties involved. The guiding principles presented in Fig. 1.1 also include commitment and equity between the different partners.

Question# 2: What are the main activities included in this life cycle–based approach?

Among the following, which is (are) true?

(A) Presubmission meetings.
(B) Submission requirements.
(C) Authorization to market.
(D) Postmarketing commitments.
(E) A reassessment of the benefit/risk ratio.
(F) All of the above are correct.

Answer: F.

(A) Presubmission meetings. They are not required for each product, but a formal meeting is available at the manufacturer's request with a regulatory agency, such as Health Canada. These meetings are not only useful during the development phase but also at the time a product is ready to be evaluated for market authorization. They are mainly intended to address questions by the manufacturer with respect to their planned drug submissions.

(B) Submission requirements. These requirements vary between product lines but refer to the efficacy and safety information required for a full evaluation of the benefit/risk ratio of the product. The requirements will also include a risk management plan (RMP) of the adverse effects associated with this medication.

(C) Authorization to market: Market authorization requires that sufficient data are available to demonstrate that the product has a favorable benefit/risk ratio. This favorable ratio should be maintained throughout the life cycle of the product. The authorization to market gives the opportunity to a regulator, such as Health Canada, FDA, EMA, and others to require the market authorization holder to conform to specific obligations throughout the process to maintain a favorable benefit/risk ratio throughout the life cycle of a product. Examples include performing pharmacoepidemiologic studies of specific populations that must be followed after the marketing authorization of the product, for example, pregnant and lactating women, children, elderly, and others.

Therefore, according to the *Food and Drug Regulations* (see Annex 1), the manufacturer is required to collect specific pharmacoepidemiologic efficacy and safety data requested at the time of marketing authorization and submit them to Health Canada and other health authorities. This information will help Health Canada and other regulatory agencies identify any changes in the benefit/risk ratio of the health product, find out if the information or instructions need to be changed or updated in the labeling of the product monograph (PM), and whether risk mitigation activities including pharmacoepidemiologic studies are required for this health product to prevent and better manage the adverse effects associated with its use (see Chapter 1, Fig. 1.1).

(D) Postmarketing commitments. This step also includes obligations that can vary according to the nature and risks associated with the health product. At this stage, there may be obligations to produce continuous passive and active surveillance of the adverse effects associated with this product (and in many cases, pharmacoepidemiologic postmarketing studies, as well as all other obligations specified at the time of initial market authorization, may be required). These obligations may be amended based on any change in the benefit/risk ratio of the product.

(E) A reassessment of the benefit/risk ratio. A reassessment based on the risk or the nature of the product may be required if necessary. The reevaluation period is determined according to the specificity of the product and can be identified as an obligation at the time of authorization to marketing. The degree of reevaluation will also be based on the product and specified in the authorization to market (see Fig. 1.1).

Supplementary Information.

Comment # 1: When a manufacturer compiles scientifically sound evidence demonstrating its health product's safety, efficacy, and quality for a specific indication (for example the treatment, mitigation, prevention, or diagnosis of a certain condition), he/she can submit the relevant information to Health Canada who will review the information included in his/her submission to appraise its compliance with the Food and Drugs Act and Regulations. If the regulator finds the information consistent with the proposed conditions of use, it will issue a notice of compliance (NOC), which includes the approval of the labeling of the product's information within the PM (see Fig. 1.1 of Chapter 1).

Comment # 2: When a manufacturer has received an NOC, the drug may then be marketed in Canada according to the specific indication that was authorized (e.g., for the treatment of this rare genetic disease mentioned in this case report). As mentioned earlier, the manufacturers must meet a number of obligations during the marketing of their product. Among these obligations, they must inform the regulatory agency of reports of serious or unexpected adverse reactions about their drug, they must follow advertising restrictions, they must update the safety guidelines for their product, and they must also maintain the quality of their drugs according to appropriate standards. In addition, all changes to the drugs after marketing authorization must be reported to Health Canada by following the appropriate guidelines and in accordance with the Food and Drugs Act and Regulations.

Comment # 3: Drugs for rare diseases, classified as orphan drugs, are often intended for serious illnesses or debilitating chronic disease. Orphan drug safety information is limited at the time of marketing due to various factors, such as the limited number of patients in clinical trials, the quality of clinical trials, and approval procedures often shorter or accelerated because of the rarity and severity of disease for which a new health product is tested.[3]

Rare diseases are an important part of public health, affecting 6%–8% of the population, and drugs for these diseases include the subcategory that has recently demonstrated marketing approval growth as new drugs in the United States.[4] In addition, considering that studies in these populations are limited by the low-disease prevalence, the natural history of the disease and the pathogenesis of the disease, in many cases, strategies commonly used for assessing the safety and efficacy known for other health products are often not applicable.

Thus, the other methodological approaches, including pharmacoepidemiologic studies of the disease history, adaptive clinical trials, metaanalysis of RCTs before marketing authorization, and the pharmacoepidemiologic studies using organized registries of patients are essential to prevent the adverse effects associated with orphan drugs. Bayesian testing and electronic databases are important strategies for the active monitoring of adverse effects related to orphan drugs[4] as discussed above.

For more information the readers are invited to consult Health Canada (2016): Regulatory Initiative: Regulations Amending the Food and Drug Regulations—Orphan Drugs—Forward Regulatory Plan 2016–18. Available at: http://www.hc-sc.gc.ca/ahc-asc/legislation/acts-reg-lois/frp-ppr/2016-2018/odrd-momr-eng.php. It is also essential to repeat that orphan drugs are also subject to the same regulatory processes concerning clinical trials and must comply with the Food and Drugs Act and Regulations. They must also comply with the ICH E6 Guidelines on Good Clinical Practice and the ICH E2A for the reporting of adverse drug reactions.

4.2 CASE REPORT # 2

4.2.1 Health Risk Management

Drug B is a monoclonal antibody inhibitor of the epidermal growth factor receptor (anti-EGFR) used for the treatment of breast cancer that has been authorized under an authorization with conditions (NOC/C). A review of the Canada Vigilance and WHO databases and other safety studies reveal significant risks of heart disorders associated with the use of drug B mainly in women presenting with the breast cancer receptor HER-2 positive; a subpopulation untested at the time of authorization for marketing (initial NDS) of drug B. The current labeling of the PM of drug B contains no information about this subpopulation of patients. Notice that the risk associated with these heart disorders appears to modify the benefit/risk ratio of drug B; measures are required to prevent the heart disorders in this subpopulation of patients and to add information to the PM to inform the health-care providers and the patients about this new risk.

Question #1: To correctly assess this risk, what general principles will you follow?

(A) Identify the problem and its context.
(B) Assess the risks and benefits.
(C) Identify and analyze options.
(D) Select a strategy.
(E) Implement the selected strategy.
(F) Monitor (supervise) and assess the results of the implementation of this strategy.
(G) All of the above are correct.

Answer: G.

To manage this problem, you can use the Health Canada risk management framework at the following link: http://www.hc-sc.gc.ca/ahc-asc/pubs/hpfb-dgpsa/risk-risques_tc-tm-eng.php. Other methods of problem solving can be used like the ones Dr. Plourde described in a recent book dealing with a difficult clinical disorder of pediatric obesity.[5]

Here, we will discuss the Health Canada model. In brief, this risk management framework consists of a series of steps, which can be grouped into three phases: the issue identification (identify the issue and its context); the assessment of risks and benefits (known and potential risks and known and potential benefits); the risk management (identify and analyze options, select strategies, implement the selected strategy, evaluate the results).

This model is flexible, in the sense that it lets you go back or move between steps or revisit steps, based on the information available. When using this model, it is important to include interested groups or affected parties, including the public and other affected parties because they play a key role in the identification of problems and assessment and management of these issues. They can provide information, knowledge, expertise, and valid insights throughout the risk management process; therefore, they should be involved as early as possible in this process of risk management.

Of course, effective risk communication is essential to ensure a proper understanding of the process by all interested groups, throughout this process. For more information on the key aspects of this model, please visit the abovementioned link or the Resources for Readers section in Annex 4.

A summary of this model includes the following six (6) steps of risk management:

(1) **Identify the problem and its context.** The purpose of this step is to clearly define and describe the problem within its relevant context. This step is critical for the risk assessment process, as it identifies the key objectives, allows us to select valid and effective strategies, and, ultimately, facilitates the allocation of available resources. The identification of the problem serves as a starting point in the process of assessment of the health risks and may be undertaken during the pre- or postapproval setting. The "context" of an issue refers to its contribution to a specific health concern, therefore, outlining its importance in relation to other problems (i.e., its priority in relation to other priorities).

↕

(2) **Assess the risks and benefits.** This step includes the assessment of health risks (known and potential) and benefits that can result from exposure to a specific agent. It also includes the evaluation of the benefit/risk assessment by weighing the risks against the benefits to determine whether the agent has a favorable benefit/risk profile. Where possible, the assessment of the risks and benefits should be performed in a multidisciplinary way, taking into account all scientifically credible information available at the time.

↕

(3) **Identify and analyze options.** With a focus on preventing risk, this step includes the identification and analysis of potential options and subsequently the formulation of a recommendation based on the most favored option. The possibilities include activities of risk management such as

change in the labeling of the PM, recall of the product by the manufacturer, and strategies for risk communication (such as letters to health-care provider, public communication, public advisory, and other types of communications). This activity places the emphasis on the following information gathering:

i. **Management of risk factors.** Recommendations regarding risk management strategies should maximize the safety of participants in clinical trials and patients in real-life situations, that is, throughout the life cycle of a health product. Other factors must also be considered such as the continuous accessibility to the product or to a valid alternative for patients. This is particularly important in situations where there is little or no alternative for the health product as in Case report # 1 above.

ii. **The nature and type of product.** For example, a biological product, as in the case presented here, which is typically available via prescription only, and under supervision/monitoring by a health-care provider, can have a risk profile and different benefits compared to an over-the-counter product (like natural health products). It should also be noted that the benefit/risk ratio linked to the use of a new chemical entity with little or no experimentation on humans may differ from the profile of a product with a well-established history on the market.

iii. **The environment in which a product is used.** For example, being exposed to a product in the experimental clinical context can generate a risk profile and different benefits in comparison to the same product administered via the special access program because it takes into account the history of the disease and the need for the subject of having access to a particular product.

iv. **Therapeutic and scientific uncertainties.** Faced with scientific uncertainty concerning the effectiveness or the validity of the therapeutic effect, the potential risk associated with the use of a product could tip the scales, such that the risks outweigh the benefit, resulting in an unfavorable benefit/risk ratio.

↕

(4) **Select a strategy.** This step is meant to improve the patient's health by minimizing the risks associated with health products. The approach recommended in the estimation of the risk management options is to consider up to four potential options, the first one being to "maintain the status quo." The three other options are chosen considering the "pros" and "cons" of each option. The recommended option should be the one in which the "pros" clearly surpass the "cons."

↕

(5) **Implement the selected strategy.** This stage includes the development and execution of a plan to implement the selected risk management

strategy. It should also include which criteria will be used to monitor and assess the effectiveness and implementation of the selected strategy.

↕

(6) Monitor (supervising) and evaluate the outcomes resulting from the implementation of this strategy. This step includes supervision of the execution of the selected risk management strategy, assessment, and recommendations for any needed changes.

Regarding drug B and the risk of cardiac disorders, the decision-making framework includes the following six (6) steps:

(1) Identify the problem and its context. As mentioned earlier, drug B was authorized according to an NOC/C and the revision of the Canada Vigilance and WHO databases as well as other pharmacoepidemiologic safety studies have revealed a significant risk of cardiac disorders associated with the use of drug B with a specific subpopulation of women with breast cancer. In short, an NOC/C provides market authorization, under the condition that the sponsor undertakes additional studies to verify the clinical benefit. For more information regarding the NOC/C, please see the following link: http://www.hc-sc.gc.ca/dhp-mps/prodpharma/applic-demande/guide-ld/compli-conform/noccg_accd-eng.php

↕

(2) Assess the risks and benefits. The revision of the safety information has raised concerns about the safety of the product and the current labeling of the PM. The risk associated with cardiac disorders in this subpopulation seems to change the benefits, creating a nonfavorable benefit/risk ratio, unless changes regarding the safety and instructions are made to the PM to prevent cardiac disorders in this subpopulation of women with breast cancer.

↕

(3) Identify and analyze options:

(A) Maintain the status quo.

(B) Require that the company carries out a pharmacoepidemiologic phase IV randomized, controlled clinical trial to assess the information on safety related to cardiac disorders in this subpopulation. This step should also include the corresponding changes to the PM to restore a positive benefit/risk ratio as prescribed by the NOC/C regulations.

(C) Require that the company carries out a pharmacoepidemiologic phase IV cohort study to evaluate the safety information about this subpopulation.

(D) Withdrawal of the product.

↕

(4) Select a strategy: Require that the company carries out a pharmacoepidemiologic phase IV randomized, controlled clinical trial to assess the information on safety related to cardiac disorders in this subpopulation.

This requirement should include the corresponding changes to the PM to restore a positive benefit/risk ratio as required by the NOC/C Guidelines. This information should be submitted in the form of a supplement to new drug submission (SNDS) to Health Canada. The other options are not acceptable; they do not represent the best interests of patients because they do not provide the best method for assessing the risk of cardiac disorders in this subpopulation of women presenting with positive HER-2 breast cancer receptors.

↕

(5) **Implementation of the selected strategy.** To ensure that all groups are involved (pre- and postmarket divisions, pharmaceutical companies, Health Care Professionals (HCPs), patient representatives, and other interested groups), a face-to-face meeting is arranged to discuss strategy and methods for implementation.

↕

(6) **Monitor (supervise) and evaluate the outcomes resulting from the implementation of this strategy:** The regulatory agency will collect the commitments made by the pharmaceutical company. It will assess their estimation of the safety information required by this randomized clinical trial. It will evaluate the new benefit/risk ratio based on the results of this new study. It will evaluate the changes made to the PM and the information provided by other documents on safety such as the RMP, educational material, and letter to health-care providers, public communications, and other types of communications.

The regulators will assess the spontaneous case reports of cardiac disorders in this subpopulation and will perform the activities of passive and active surveillance such as the review of the development safety update report (DSUR), the periodic benefit–risk evaluation report (PBRER), and other pharmacoepidemiologic safety studies, to ensure that the strategy chosen led to a significant reduction in the number of reported cases of cardiac disorders in this subpopulation.

4.3 CASE REPORT # 3

4.3.1 Risk Assessment and Safety Measures

A 56-year-old patient with colon cancer and metastasis to the liver for 2 years started a treatment with drug C 3 months ago studied in combination with drug D. The patient received three doses of the drug C and drug D in a combination regimen while in the study; the most recent administration was on July 24, 2014, which is prior to the beginning of the adverse effect.

On August 15, 2014, a magnetic resonance imaging (MRI) with and without contrast was performed. The test revealed specific changes on the patient's brain white matter. It is important to note that this observation could also result from previous chemotherapy treatments, which are also associated with changes on brain white matter. It is unlikely that the changes seen with the MRI are atypical of a neoplastic process.

At the beginning of the study, the initial MRI of the patient's brain had revealed no evidence of metastatic disease or other abnormalities. The patient also has a medical history of hypertension and type 2 diabetes mellitus. Note that the same adverse event has been observed among other participants in this study.

Question #1: With the help of the Naranjo algorithm to assess causality, what is your assessment?

(A) Certain >9;
(B) Probable 5–8;
(C) Possible 1–4;
(D) Unlikely 0.

Answer: C.

According to the algorithm of Naranjo (https://livertox.nih.gov/Naranjoassessment.pdf) an adverse event is possibly drug-related if we consider that we have previous conclusive reports outlining this reaction with the drugs in the study (+1) and that there is a temporal relationship between this event and the administration of these drugs (+2).

To further support the relationship, the investigator noted that, when the patient began to take the drugs in the study, an initial brain MRI had not demonstrated any specific (+1) changes.

During the last months, the patient also developed language abnormalities and had equilibrium problems but not of other focal findings, which adds weight to the objective conclusions advocating that there is a causal link between the changes observed in the brain white matter and the fact of taking the drugs under study. In addition, the symptoms disappeared when the drugs were discontinued (+1).

There are other possible explanations, including the presence of hypertension and type 2 diabetes mellitus (−1). Considering that we do not have any other information on this case, we will assess it as being possibly related to the drugs under study.

Supplementary Information.

Comment # 1 Note that D is an antiangiogenic, authorized in Canada, and as for other antiangiogenic in the same class, there is a potential risk of embolic arterial incident, bleeding, and hypertension after intravenous administration of this class of health product. Should we suspect a role of D in this case? This certainly deserves a follow-up with pharmacoepidemiologic studies to assess whether or not there is a difference when C is used as monotherapy, in comparison to its use in combination with drug D.

Comment # 2 Based on the case report, it is difficult to be convinced of the reasons for the changes in the white matter. We believe that most of the anomalies measured with the MRI in this 56-year-old patient are vascular in origin and their increase is common with age. In addition, these abnormalities may also be associated with concurrent comorbidities such as diabetes mellitus, arteriosclerosis, and hypertension. Note that our patient has a history of high blood pressure and type 2 diabetes mellitus that could explain these anomalies.

Question #2: Which of these would require ensuring that the benefit/risk ratio remains positive?

(A) A monitoring plan.
(B) A comprehensive assessment of similar cases.
(C) A constant follow-up of this case and other cases, as required.
(D) A comprehensive assessment of the benefit/risk ratio.
(E) All of the above.

Answer: E.

(A) A monitoring plan. With respect to our adverse drug reaction, it would be good to require that all patients who participate in studies with drug C undergo brain MRI with and without contrast on registration in the study and during subsequent routine testing. This monitoring plan must also include frequent neurological examinations by the attending physician and a plan to stop the treatment and follow-up after treatment for patients with clinical reactions and/or clinically significant radiological images to identify and treat patients at risk and at an early stage of the disease.

(B) A comprehensive assessment of similar cases. A total of 128 patients, who had been treated with drug C, underwent initial tests with brain MRI. Among them, we identified six patients with a new signal. Due to the high prevalence of signals on the MRI in the population of $\geq$50 years old, it is difficult for the moment to certify whether the findings are related to treatment with drug C or D or due to a normal aging process or to the previous patient's medical history. On the other hand, it is required that the sponsor of these clinical trials continues to follow closely the participants in pharmacoepidemiology clinical studies and produce a complete assessment of similar cases to ensure the safety of participants in these clinical trials (see also C and D).

(C) A constant follow-up of this case and other cases, as required. Until we have sufficient information, the sponsor must continue to follow the known cases of this adverse drug reaction and document any other new case as medically important incidents and report these cases to regulatory agencies promptly to conform to the requirements of section C.05.014 (1) Part C—Division 5 of the Food and Drugs Regulations (see Annex 1, below) and the ICH E2A and ICH E6 Guidelines available at the Resources for Readers section (Annex 4).

(D) A comprehensive assessment of the benefit/risk ratio. According to Part C, Division 1 of the Food and Drug Regulations, the manufacturer shall provide to the Minister, in the form of a summary report, all information related to an adverse reaction to a drug at national and international level, on an annual basis or on request (see above), if there are problems related to the safety of a drug to comply with articles C.01.018 and C.01.019 of this regulation, respectively (see Annex 1 below).

Supplementary Information.

Comment # 3 As this drug is not approved in any country, we request an assessment of the benefit/risk ratio for this product in the form of a DSUR because it includes an analysis of the safety for the drugs in development with an estimate of the benefit/risk ratio from clinical trials.

Question #3: How would you require the risk to be communicated to ensure the safety of participants in clinical trials?

(A) Update the investigator's brochure (IB).
(B) Update the protocol.
(C) Update the consent form.
(D) Update the PM.
(E) A, B, and C are true.
(F) All of the above are true.

Answer: E.

(A) Update the IB. According to Part C, Division 5 of the Food and Drug Regulations, for drugs intended for clinical trials on human subjects: the "IB" refers, in what concerns a drug, to a document containing the preclinical and clinical data on the drug described in the next paragraph C.05.005 (e): the IB contains the following information:

(i) physical, chemical, and pharmaceutical properties of drugs;
(ii) the pharmacological aspects of the drug, including its metabolites observed in the animal species tested;
(iii) the pharmacokinetics of the drug behavior and metabolism, including how it is biologically transformed in the tested animal species;
(iv) if applicable, the toxicological effects of the drug observed in animal species tested in studies in single dose, repeated dose, or special studies;
(v) as appropriate, the results of studies of carcinogenicity in animal species tested for the drug;
(vi) where appropriate, the results of clinical studies on the pharmacokinetics of the drug;
(vii) conduct as appropriate, when clinical trials have already been completed on human subjects, the following information obtained during these tests: safety of drugs, its pharmacodynamic behavior, its effectiveness, and its dose responses;
(viii) if the drug is a radioactive pharmaceutical product within the meaning of article C.03.201, information on the mode of product preparation as well as for the prepared product radiation dosimetry and the storage conditions.

The IB should be reviewed at least annually and revised, if necessary, in accordance with the sponsor's written procedures. A more frequent revision may be appropriate, depending on the stage of development and the amount of new information generated. However, according to the ICH E6 Guidelines, the new relevant information may be significant enough to be communicated to researchers and possibly to the institutional review boards, the independent ethic committees and/or regulatory authorities, including Health Canada, before including it in the form of a revised IB.

Thus, in addition to including this new information in the IB, instructions will be provided to researchers regarding the identification, treatment, and follow-up of patients with this adverse effect, even if the research project has been discontinued. See the ICH E6 Guidelines on Good Clinical Practice to supplement the obligations and the content of this IB information. The aim is to protect the participants in clinical trials against all new adverse effect associated with taking the drug(s) in question.

(B) Update the Protocol. "Protocol" described in the document sets out the objectives, work plan, methodology, statistical considerations, and organization of a clinical trial. Considering that a monitoring plan will be added to this adverse effect, it should be clearly stipulated in the protocol to warn all researchers of such changes and to comply with the Food and Drugs Act and Regulations.

(C) Update the consent form. A consent form is a process whereby a given patient confirms voluntarily that he or she is willing to participate in a particular trial, after having been duly informed of all aspects of the trial and of its adverse effects, which may influence the decision about participating. Informed consent is documented in writing, signed, and dated on the informed consent form. Considering the information discussed above concerning the adverse effect it is pretty relevant that the adverse effect must be clearly written in the consent form, in a language accessible to the participants to ensure that the patient makes an informed decision about his/her participation in clinical trials in accordance with the Food and Drug Regulations.

(D) Update the PM. Because this product is not marketed in Canada or other countries, no PM is available. Therefore, no update to this document can be performed at this time. However, if the sponsor wishes to submit an NDS to evaluate this product for the purpose of receiving marketing authorization, it must also provide an original PM containing the required information. For more information on the content and format of the PM, the readers are invited to consult the following link: http://www.hc-sc.gc.ca/dhp-mps/prodpharma/applic-demande/guide-ld/label_guide_ld-eng.php; please note that information associated with the adverse effect should be provided in this document.

Any new safety information obtained as a result of the marketing authorization of this product should also be included in the PM and communicated to health-care providers and the public, if necessary, in the form of letters to the health-care providers, hospitals, and the public. Because the product is not marketed, such letters are not required, but the IB, research protocol, and consent form will need to be updated to ensure the safety of the participants in these clinical trials.

4.4 CASE REPORT # 4

4.4.1 Biosimilar Biological Drug and its Surveillance

This case report concerns drug E for which an authorization application to market as a biosimilar biological drug (BBD) based on data from the reference biological product (RBP) (drug F) has been filed. Note that drug F is not authorized in Canada, but it is authorized in Europe.

Drug E is an identical product with identical contents, in terms of excipients and concentration, and it is considered similar to drug F with regard to the quality requirements. Drug E is administered via subcutaneous infusion at a dose and frequency comparable to health product F. Drug F is a monoclonal antibody that blocks the tumor necrosis factor alpha (TNFα), a key human tumor inflammatory cytokine involved in the pathogenesis of several inflammatory diseases. Drug F is licensed for six (6) indications and is used in patients who have inflammatory diseases. Specific diseases for which drug F is authorized in adults are rheumatoid arthritis (RA), ankylosing spondylitis (AS), Crohn's disease (CD), and ulcerative colitis (UC). It is also authorized in pediatrics for indications of CD and UC. On the basis of a reduced nonclinical and clinical data bank, the promoter requested a marketing authorization for drug E that would include all the information and uses currently allowed for drug F. Comparative repetitive dose toxicity studies in rats revealed that drug E and drug F were comparable in terms of pharmacological doses and toxicological and toxicokinetics effects. Pharmacodynamic (PD) and pharmacokinetic (PK) studies have also demonstrated that drug E cannot be distinguished from the drug F, based on various selected PD and PK parameters. The sponsor has submitted a phase III study of safety and efficacy to support the absence of significant clinical difference between drugs E and F. The phase III study on safety and efficacy was conducted on adult patients with RA, whereas the PK study was conducted on adult patients with active SA. No clinical study has tested the product on patients with the other inflammatory diseases mentioned above (CD and UC). Therefore, concerning these other inflammatory diseases, the approval for those indications and uses need an extrapolation from the clinical studies already submitted. The proposed PM for drug E study is identical to the PM for drug F.

Question #1: Which of the following studies are desirable?

(A) Preclinical studies.
(B) Comparative PKs and PDs studies.

(C) Studies used to assess efficacy and safety.
(D) An RMP must also be submitted.
(E) All these studies are desirable.

Answer: E.

(A) Preclinical studies. Preclinical toxicity studies show that drug E is well tolerated in animals. However, changes were observed at the subcutaneous injection sites, which is common with drugs injected by this route. If drug E is authorized for marketing, it should be recommended to participants, during clinical trials and patients in the postapproval marketing phase, that the injection sites are rotated on a daily basis to reduce local risks associated with the injection. In conclusion, the information provided by the sponsor from the preclinical studies is adequate to assess the safety profile of drug E and to support its use in humans, provided that appropriate safety precautions are taken, including the rotation of the injection sites during the use of the drug.

If the product is authorized for marketing, these safety precautions will need to be added to the PM by following the specific guidelines. Thus, the manufacturer shall develop a PM for the BBDs in accordance with the principles, practices, and processes presented in the Guidelines on BBDs and on PM guidance documents (see Annex 4, Resources for Readers).

(B) Comparative PKs and PDs studies. The sponsor has conducted a bioavailability study to characterize the PK parameters of drug E and comparative PK and PD studies of drug F. These comparative PK and PD studies were led on healthy adults. Based on the data submitted by the sponsor, PK and PD parameters are comparable between drugs E and F: the PK study demonstrated satisfactory comparability for the indication of AS.

Thus, these studies show bioavailability and bioequivalence between drugs E and F. For more information on comparative bioavailable studies, the reader is invited to consult the following link: Guidance Document: Conduct and Analysis of Comparative Bioavailability Studies. http://www.hc-sc.gc.ca/dhp-mps/prodpharma/applic-demande/guide-ld/bio/gd_cbs_ebc_ld-eng.php.

(C) Studies used to assess effectiveness and safety. The conclusion of this phase III study is that efficacy and safety are very similar between drugs E and F. In summary, the sponsor responded positively to the requirements to assess the efficacy and safety of drug E.

(D) An RMP must also be submitted. According to the Guidelines for manufacturers (requirements for information and submission to BBDs that can be found at the Resources for Readers section), it is important that an RMP is presented before granting of a marketing authorization for drug E. The RMP should be designed to track and detect both known and potential issues related to efficacy and safety of drug E that may have an impact on the benefit/risk ratio of these BBDs. For more information on the surveillance and intervention activities in postapproval marketing phase, the reader can refer to Chapter 1, Fig. 1.1.

Question #2: Which of the following considerations are essential to remember?

(A) Considerations related to labeling.
(B) Considerations related to the notion of substitutions.
(C) Considerations related to the interchangeability.
(D) Considerations related to extrapolation to other indications.
(E) Considerations related to the traceability of the side effects.
(F) All of these considerations are essential.

Answer: F.

(A) Considerations related to labeling. The labeling of drug E must be different and not a copy of drug F as presented here. The promoter of a BBD cannot use the PM of the RBP in its entirety for his own product. The development requires a PM for the BBDs, which is in accordance with the principles, practices, and processes presented in the Guidelines for BBDs and concerning the PM available at the Resources for Readers section.

(B) Considerations related to the notion of substitutions. Because of the differences between the BBD and the RBP and potential risks that may arise, the pharmacist should not proceed to a substitution of one product by another. These differences are also true between different BBDs to a same RBP. In conclusion, the substitution of an RBP by BBDs or vice versa may expose the patient to unexpected clinical consequences and is therefore not recommended to ensure the safety of patients.[6]

(C) Considerations related to the interchangeability. When products are interchangeable, it means that the BBD is biologically similar to the RBP and that it will produce the same clinical results as the RBP in any patient. In addition, if the product must be administered more than once, the risk of reduction of efficacy and change of safety in alternating BBDs/RBP profile should be the same as if the RBP was repeatedly administered without alternating with the BBD.[6] Interchangeability, however, is not without risk; it is the responsibility of the physician to decide for the best interests of patients.

From the scientific and medical point of view, biological products, without regard to their status of RBP or BBD, should not be interchangeable in absence of strong clinical data. In Canada, the notion of interchangeability is the responsibility of the health-care system, which is under the responsibility of the provinces and territories. Health Canada is not in favor of interchangeability of a reference biological product (RBP) for its BBD and recommends that doctors take perfectly informed decisions about therapeutic interchangeability.[6]

(D) Considerations related to extrapolation to other indications. If the therapeutic similarity is demonstrated for an indication, it could be extrapolated to other indications of the RBP in case the mechanism of action of the BBDs is dependent on its interaction with a target (i.e., only one connection is possible). It is also important to note that the risk of adverse effects might be different for a product depending on its therapeutic indication.

In Canada, the criteria used for the extrapolation of the data to the BBDs require the demonstration of similarity between the RBP and the BBDs by an overall comparison of the two products. Also consider that even when the two products are generally comparable, minor and generally unimportant differences between two active ingredients may affect the mechanism of action; in this case, extrapolation is excluded.[6]

Also note that differences in the physiopathological mechanism of the disease (indications and uses) prevent the extrapolation and this is true both for the BBDs and generic products.[6] Because the pathophysiology of inflammatory diseases of the intestine (CD and UC) is different from that of rheumatoid disease (RD) (the patient populations), an extrapolation to RD and AS to CD and UC cannot be recommended due to the absence of specific clinical PK and PD studies. In addition, the safety profile is different between rheumatic diseases and inflammatory diseases of the intestine, and this, for the whole class of TNFα inhibitors.

In particular, the risk of hepatosplenic lymphoma in adolescents and young adults appears only if that product is associated with inflammatory diseases of the intestine; taking this into consideration, extrapolation of findings to these indications is unacceptable.

(E) Considerations related to the traceability of the side effects. The passive and active surveillance activities of adverse effects following the marketing of BBDs should ensure the traceability of the adverse effects associated with these new products. In addition to the challenges mentioned regarding the surveillance of adverse effects associated with health products in general, the BBDs pose additional challenges. Therefore, we need to find ways for the follow-up of the adverse effects associated with these drugs such as providing information on the brand name and the lot number of the drug to trace them.

Question #3: Which of the following are true?

(A) The RBP is a major element.
(B) The BBDs are subject to the same regulatory requirements as the RBPs.
(C) There must be a similarity between the RBP and the BBDs.
(D) All of the above are true.

Answer: D.

(A) The RBP is a major element. The concept of BBD applies to all biological drug submissions for which the promoter is seeking marketing authorization, based on a similarity with an already approved RBP.[6] This application relies in part on existing data about the RBP to submit a reduced set of clinical and nonclinical data in the NDS process. The RBP is the essential element in the process of development and marketing authorization of the BBDs.[6]

The RBP is the product to which a BBD is compared in studies that will establish similarity of the two products. To be considered an RBP, the biological health product must first be authorized in the light of a thorough assessment of a complete set of data on the quality, nonclinical and clinical data.[6]

(B) The BBDs are subject to the same regulatory requirements as the RBPs. The BBDs are subject to the same regulations as the RBPs, which means that the manufacturer of the BBDs must conform to Part C of Division 8 of the Food and Drugs Regulations including sections C.08.002, C.08.002 (2) and C.08.004 (1) (a) (1) that describe the requirements associated with the NDS. In the case of BBDs, manufacturers must submit an NDS for review purposes, which will provide a basis for their application to market, although the extent of the clinical data required may be different or reduced, compared to that required for the RBP.[6]

In addition to the rigorous approval process implemented before approval of the BBDs, which takes into account issues related to the safety of participants in clinical trials, BBD manufacturers will have to provide a detailed RMP on how their product-related safety issues will be managed and monitored in postapproval marketing, in accordance with the concept of product life cycle.

Supplementary Information.

Comment # 1 When the BBD has obtained an NOC, it is considered a new biological drug, i.e., a "full" product, and is covered by all regulatory requirements applicable to biological products. Thus, all the laws and all the principles set out in the Food and Drugs Act and Regulations including data protection, the patented medicines (NOC), the Patent Act, and Intellectual Property apply to the BBDs. On the other hand, a BBD cannot be used for another presentation of BBDs.

As in the case of innovative products, with the development of the BBDs, companies must demonstrate that their products meet the quality standards required for all biological products. Thus, they must respect the Good Laboratory Practice, Good Manufacturing Practice, and Good Clinical Practice Guidelines (see Resources for Readers section) for both the RBPs and the BBDs.

However, by using existing information from the public domain concerning the RBP, manufacturers reduce the duration in the development of the BBDs, which will also have an impact on the reduction of costs associated with their production.[6]

Comment # 2 The clinical studies conducted in Canada and involving the BBDs are subject to Part C, Division 5 of The Food and Drug Regulations (see Annex 3), which describe the provisions applying to clinical trials on human subjects in Canada. Clinical trial applications should be presented in a way that meets the Health Canada Clinical Trials Guidelines.

In their application for authorization, the sponsor must include all the information specified in section C.05.005 of the Food and Drug Regulations. If an RBP to Canada is used in the context of clinical trials conducted in Canada, the manufacturer must provide data to validate the safety of the drug and those must meet the requirements of RBPs.

(C) There must be a similarity between the RBP and the BBDs. To establish the similarity between the BBD and the chosen RBP, the manufacturer must conduct a comparability exercise. Comparability analyses are done in three phases, namely:

- **i.** the comparability in terms of quality to the physicochemical characteristics (molecular composition of the active substance and its impurities) and biological properties (functional activity and ability to produce the desired effect);
- **ii.** the pharmacological comparability (analyses in vitro, for example, binding to receptors or tests based on the cells as well as PD studies on in vivo models) (in appropriate animals);
- **iii.** the clinical comparability (comparative PK and PD studies followed by comparative efficacy and safety studies). The nonclinical and clinical requirements for the approval of the BBDs are generally more limited compared to those for the approval of the RBP because it relies partly on data from the RBP.
- **iv.** The assessment is mainly based on data from comparative studies between the RBP and the BBDs, according to a short program. Abbreviated clinical trials help not only to avoid unnecessary testing in humans but also to reduce the development costs associated with clinical trials.

Question #4: This submission must be rejected because the comparator is not authorized in Canada.

True or false.

Answer: False.

According to the Guidelines, in some cases, the manufacturer may use an RBP that is not authorized in Canada.[6] To do this, the manufacturer must demonstrate that it complies with the following conditions:

- **i.** the presentation should include enough information to explain in detail the link between the two products and should confirm that the two products are marketed by the same pharmaceutical company for innovative biological products or by the same company that has received approval to market the medicinal ingredient in the same pharmaceutical form as that in Canada;
- **ii.** the sponsor shall ensure that the RBP in Canada is associated with sufficient information and data to support the submission;
- **iii.** the RBP in Canada must come from a country that has established links with the regulatory body responsible for reviewing this submission and this is acceptable with Europe;
- **iv.** the use of the RBP in Canada is marketed on a large scale in a country that officially joined the ICH Guidelines and which has regulatory

standards, guidelines for drug evaluation, monitoring postmarketing, and an approach of comparability similar to what occurs in Canada;

v. if the RBP in Canada is used in Canadian clinical trials, data must be provided to satisfy the chemistry and manufacturing requirements under section C.05.005 of the Food and Drugs Regulations; and finally

vi. the sponsor must contact the regulatory agency early in the drug development process to verify that the RBP is appropriate. Because these conditions are met by sponsor, it would be wrong to reject this submission based on the fact that the RBP is not authorized in Canada.

Question #5: No indication can be extrapolated in absence of data supporting this indication in a submission.

True or false.

Answer: False.

According to the Guidelines, any claim made by the promoter of the BBDs must be supported by appropriate scientific data, which would normally include data on safety and efficacy obtained with the BBDs. However, sometimes presentations relating to additional information held by the RBP can be granted to the BBDs in the absence of such clinical data.

In some cases, the presentation of comparative PK and PD data to make the bridge between two or more indications may be sufficient. It may also be possible to extrapolate clinical data for other indications when the reasons are persuasive and well-documented scientifically.

The extrapolation should be justified based on: (1) the mechanism of action of the product, (2) the physiopathological mechanism of disease or the disorders in question, (3) the safety profile of the conditions and/or respective populations, and (4) clinical experiences related to the RBP.

A detailed scientific justification that adequately addresses the benefits and risks of this presentation should be provided to support adequately the extrapolation of the data. Thus, it is acceptable (on a case-by-case basis) to extrapolate an indication from a different population, from the data of a different population with this same indication. For more information, please see the BBDs Guidelines at the Resources for Readers section.

4.5 CASE REPORT # 5

4.5.1 Rare Diseases and How to Deal with a Small Number of Patients

The rare hereditary disease we deal with now is associated with mutations at the level of a gene that encodes for a specific protein. These mutations cause an uncontrolled increase in certain inflammatory cytokines, which are considered to be responsible for the clinical manifestations and the pathology of this orphan idiopathic inflammatory disease made up of four autosomal dominant disorders. Each disorder shares several common recurring symptoms such as fever/chills, arthralgia, fatigue, and other symptoms. Symptoms usually appear in late childhood or early adolescence. It is estimated that 25 to 40 patients are affected by this disease in Canada, which fits very well with the definition of an orphan disease. There is no approved therapy available in Canada for this rare inherited disease.

Drug H is a humanized monoclonal antibody genetically modified that blocks the activity of these inflammatory cytokines, with high affinity. It is the first product in its class, suggested for the treatment of patients with this disease in Canada. The promoter is looking for a marketing authorization for the drug to deal with this rare disease in adults and children 9 years and older. Data submitted on efficacy from several countries provide sufficient evidence to assert that drug H is effective in reducing the signs and symptoms in patients with this disease.

Safety data currently available suggest that the risks associated with the drug are manageable as long as safety measures are implemented to facilitate the identification and treatment of adverse effects associated with this therapy. Therefore, the benefit/risk ratio is considered acceptable.

Question #1: What are the restrictions associated with the study of orphan diseases?

(A) The restrictions include the fact that there is no formal regulatory guidance for the investigator in the clinical assessment of these diseases.
(B) There are little or no prespecific clinical practice guidelines on the management of this disease.
(C) Considering the small number of subjects involved in the clinical trials, the efficacy and safety information is rather limited.
(D) All of the above are true.

Answer: D.

(A) The restrictions include the fact that there is no formal regulatory guidance for the investigator in the clinical assessment of these diseases: Health Canada is currently developing an approach to appoint, approve, and track the orphan medical products to make them beneficial for Canadians with rare diseases, but currently, there is no formal regulatory guidance for investigators in the clinical assessment of these diseases.

This new structure retains the current requirements based on clinical trials and will be supported by an intensified exchange of information between international partners. Approved drugs will be continuously kept under surveillance to ensure their efficacy and safety through their life cycle.

(B) There are little or no prespecific clinical practice guidelines on the management of this disease: The estimation and evaluation of the seriousness of this disease in these patients are guided by the doctor's clinical judgment and knowledge of the medical history of the patient who, accordingly, is subject to interpretation. As mentioned, most of the time, there is no available clinical practice guideline on rare or orphan diseases that can lead to a lack of compatibility between the researchers and doctors in the evaluation of these diseases.

(C) Considering the small number of subjects involved in the clinical trials, the efficacy and safety information is rather limited: Considering that we are dealing with a rare disease, clinical studies were conducted from small sample sizes, especially in the pediatric population. There were no controlled study, placebo, or other about the four different types of genotype associated with this disease. However, this is acceptable in the case of diseases for which no therapy is authorized. In addition, data on the efficacy and safety in the long-term use of drug H in the treatment of this disease are limited.

Obviously, cumulative reports on the efficacy, safety, and the PK data on present studies and a registry of patients for the drug will be required. For more information the reader is invited to consult Health Canada (2016): Regulatory Initiative: Regulations Amending the Food and Drug Regulations—Orphan Drugs—Forward Regulatory Plan 2016–18. Available at: http://www.hc-sc.gc.ca/ahc-asc/legislation/acts-reg-lois/frp-ppr/2016-2018/odrd-momr-eng.php.

Question #2: What should we consider to ensure that we have maintained a favorable benefit/risk ratio when the product has been authorized?

(A) Submit detailed information about all adverse reactions including infections, immunogenicity, hepatotoxicity reactions, and others produced during all trials with drug H.

(B) Submit, in the form of an SNDS, all study reports related to the efficacy and the long-term safety of drug H in the treatment of this disease.

(C) Submit, in the form of an SNDS, all study reports pertaining to drug H analyzed by phenotypes.

(D) Submit the data used in the assessment of the benefit/risk ratio including data collected in other jurisdictions (FDA, EMA, and others).

(E) Provide the pharmacovigilance plan for the adverse effects associated with drug H: including the PBRERs, the RMP, the DSUR, and others, as well as all updates to the PM of drug H.

(F) Provide all reports and correspondence submitted by other jurisdictions, including the follow-up commitments, obligations in postapproval marketing, and others.

(G) Provide a registry for Canadian patients who receive drug H, immediately after the issuance of the NOC, the plan for the registry, and the registration procedures.

(H) All of the above are true.

Answer: H.

As for all other health products, reports of adverse events should be submitted to conform with section C.01.017 of the Food and Drug Regulations: The manufacturer shall submit to the minister a report of all information related to the following serious adverse drug reactions within 15 days after receiving or becoming aware of the information, whichever occurs first:

(a) any serious adverse drug reaction that has occurred in Canada with respect to the drug;
(b) any serious unexpected adverse drug reaction that has occurred outside Canada with respect to the drug.

Each unexpected serious adverse reaction that is subject to an expedited report must be reported individually, in accordance with section C.05.014 of the Food and Drug Regulations and in accordance with the ICH E2A Guidelines on clinical safety data management: definitions and standards for expedited reporting that can be found at the Resources for Readers section.

Because it is an orphan disease, the plan for the program and the procedures for entry in the registry for Canadian patients who receive drug H must be provided to the regulatory agency and includes:

(1) all reports and correspondence regarding the registry program;
(2) regular safety and efficacy data from the registry for adults and children;
(3) the list of patients who withdrew from clinical studies and their records, with the dates and reasons for withdrawal and other related information.

Whereas the clinical studies in these populations are limited by a low prevalence of these diseases, strategies commonly used for the assessment of safety and efficacy in the postapproval marketing phase such as postmarket metaanalysis and spontaneous reports on adverse reactions are only minimally applicable.

Therefore other methodological approaches, including pharmacoepidemiologic studies of the natural history of the disease, the appropriate clinical trials, metaanalysis of RCTs before marketing authorization, and epidemiological studies using patient registries, are essential for the prevention of adverse effects in the case of orphan drugs.

Bayesian analysis and electronic databases are important strategies for active monitoring of adverse effects associated with orphan drugs. For more information regarding the active and passive surveillance of adverse drug reactions, the reader is invited to review previous sections of this book.

4.6 CASE REPORT # 6

4.6.1 Pharmacoepidemiologic Studies and Related Considerations

Drug I is a humanized monoclonal antibody that selectively binds and neutralizes the biological activity of the vascular endothelial growth factor (anti-VEGF). It is authorized in Canada, the United States, and Europe for the treatment of breast and colon cancers. For colon cancer, drug I is authorized at a dose of 200 mg per day, whereas for breast cancer the dose is 400 mg twice per day. Each year, thousands of patients are treated with drug I, worldwide. Since 2010, more than 60 case reports describing the occurrence of intracranial hemorrhage have been reported after the use of drug I. Affected patients are primarily women between 45 and 70 years old, who used drug I in the treatment of breast cancer. Between January 2006 and January 2016, 44 spontaneous reports of intracranial bleeding associated with drug I in breast cancer (32 cases) and colon cancer (12 cases) have been reported. These cases were evaluated by the manufacturer as being probably related to use of drug I by the Naranjo algorithm (see the Case Report # 3). In response to the concerns about these spontaneous case reports, a comparative observational study about events of intracranial bleeding with drug I, composed of men and women between 45 and 70 years, has been set up. The study is designed to evaluate the association between intracranial hemorrhages and the use of drug I in the cases of breast and colon cancers. Intracranial hemorrhages were diagnosed based on clinical symptoms and/or subarachnoid bleeding signs seen on brain computer tomography (CT) or on brain MRI or by the presence of xanthochromia on lumbar puncture.

The eligibility criteria for patients include the ages between 45 and 70, a complete interview within 30 days following the episode of intracranial bleeding to reduce the possibility of recall bias; the absence of a prior history of brain injury that might increase the risk of bleeding such as an arterial–venous malformation, a tumor, or an aneurysm, and the absence of prior history of intracranial bleeding. Due to the mechanism of action of drug I, patients treated with this product are at higher risk of bleeding. According to the available documentation, the frequency of intracranial bleeding is 0.6 cases per million populations annually around the world.

Question #1: Among the following pharmacoepidemiologic studies, which should you favor?

(A) RCT.
(B) Prospective cohort study.
(C) Case-control study.

Answer: C.

(A) Randomized controlled trial (RCT). RCTs have the advantage of producing information that is less impacted by biases (higher internal validity). RCT presents a forward-looking experiment in which patients are assigned, at random, to be exposed or not exposed to the drug tested. The two groups are evaluated based on the appearance or not of the event of interest whether they are exposed to the drug tested or not. However, RCTs are not always possible due to the ethical implications of assigning a potentially harmful exposure to a group of patients (see also Case Report #8 below). Therefore, A is not the best answer.

(B) Prospective cohort study includes following a predefined cohort of patients over time. After a set follow-up period, the exposed group and unexposed groups can be compared to determine whether there is a greater risk of developing the adverse event of interest in the exposed versus unexposed group. These studies provide a substitute to RCTs in cases where an RCT is not logically or ethically feasible.

When the events of interest studied are rare, too much time and too many resources would be required to demonstrate significant trends in a prospective cohort study. Therefore, B is not the best answer. However, note that had a retrospective cohort study been available, this would have been a feasible alternative.

(C) Case-control study involves two groups: one with the event of interest and one without this event of interest, selected by researchers who assess retrospectively the presence or the absence of exposure to a causative agent. When the event of interest is rare or takes a long time to develop, this kind of study is particularly useful. Here the event of interest (intracranial hemorrhages) is rare, which makes the case-control study very interesting. Because an RCT or a prospective cohort study is not possible due to ethical concerns and/or logistics, the best answer is C.

Please notice that the presence of similar comparison groups is necessary because it has a great influence on the credibility of the results. With these three models of studies, it is possible to create similar comparison groups with regard to their baseline characteristics. For more information on the comparison groups, the reader is invited to consult the ICH E10 Guidelines, which is listed in the Resources for Readers section below.

Supplementary Information.

Comment #1 A case-control study involves selecting the cases first. For example, to know if exposure to X increases the risk of Y, we select a group of patients with Y disease first. Once we have selected the cases, the controls are selected (similar patients but who do not have the disease Y), then retrospectively, we go back to see which cases and controls were exposed to X. Then we can calculate an odds ratio (OR) to see if the odds of being exposed to X were greater in the cases versus the controls.

On the other hand, in a retrospective case study, we identify a cohort of patients that have been followed over time for another purpose, some of these patients will have the disease Y and others will not. Then we retrospectively go back to assess their exposure at the time the cohort was initially created and then identify who, at this point in time, has the disease.

This is different from a prospective cohort study where we would gather the cohort from the beginning, based on exposure and follow them into the future. In brief, in case control studies, the cases are identified first, and exposure is assessed retrospectively, whereas in cohort studies, the cases are identified over time, prospectively.

Question #2: To which of the following questions should you pay attention?

(A) What is the similarity between the comparison groups?
(B) Were the exposure and outcomes measured in the same way between the compared groups?
(C) What is the strength of the association between exposure and outcome?
(D) What is the accuracy of the estimated risk?
(E) What is the magnitude of the risk (i.e., its clinical importance)?
(F) Should the clinical practice be changed because of the results of this study?
(G) All of the above are true.

Answer: G.

(A) What is the similarity between the comparison groups? This issue greatly influences the credibility of the results. Ideally, the comparison groups should be totally similar except from the point of view of the exposure in RCTs and in cohort studies and for the event of interest in case-control studies. RCT are theoretically the best studies to ensure the homogeneity of the comparison groups in regards to the different determinants of a known or unknown result (with the exception of the exposure).

Given the observational nature of cohorts and case-control studies, it is very important that these studies be conducted with predetermined exclusion/inclusion criteria to ensure that the subjects in the study are similar with respect to their baseline characteristics. It is therefore very important that researchers carefully document the characteristics of the two comparison groups and demonstrate their similarity or statistical control for their differences. Some of the characteristic differences between the groups may represent confounding factors.

Even if the researchers control the confounding factors or demonstrate their equivalence in both groups, an imbalance can occur between other confounding factors of which the researchers are not aware and which can influence the outcome.

(B) Were the exposure and outcomes measured in the same way between the compared groups? Case-control studies are subject to recall bias, investigator bias, and selection bias in the evaluation of exposure. Investigators may use strategies to minimize these biases to ensure, for example, that the assumptions of the study are not known either by the investigators and or by the subjects (double blind).

Exposure should be measured the same way for the case and the controls, otherwise the real risk might be different from what is reported by the study: higher if the controls were most at risk, lower if the controls were less exposed. In our example, exposure was measured in the same way in the cases and controls. As mentioned, case-control studies in general are sensitive to some recall bias and investigator bias.

We can prevent the recall bias by using a very structured interview when the subjects do not know the assumptions and are questioned shortly after the event in question.

In our example, a complete interview was conducted within 30 days following the episode of intracranial hemorrhage, which is acceptable. Several strategies can be used to reduce the possibility of selection bias including the monitoring of active cases and the determination of objective eligibility criteria.

(C) How strong is the association between exposure and outcome? The strength of the association will always be lessened for cohorts and case-control studies because of the possibility of having confounding factors for which statistical adjustment has not been performed. The relative risk (RR) is the most common way to express the relationship between exposure and consequence in RCT and cohort studies.

The OR is used in the case-control studies. When the event of interest is uncommon, as observed here in the population for which the sample has been taken, the OR approaches of the RR.

The strength of the association will be lower in this kind of study because the case-control model that is used with some confounding factors could not be recognized. In this study, the OR is very high (which suggests a strong association) for the indication of breast cancer with regard to the relationship between drug I and intracranial hemorrhage. As shown below, the OR is of 9.98 with a confidence interval (CI) at 95% of 5.5−14.2 with a probability of $P = .02$.

The strength of the relationship appears high and significant among women who used drug I for all indications, combined with OR of 2.00, a CI 95%: 1.00−4.00, and a probability of $P < .05$. However, there is no significant association between drug I and the intracranial bleeding in women with colon cancer.

Therefore, it is possible to believe that the association between drug I and intracranial hemorrhage in women is the result of the strong association between the use of drug I and breast cancer. The association did not prove to be significant for the use of drug I regarding colon cancer in men.

You can use a 2×2 contingency table to calculate the OR;

According to the following equation: $OR = (a/c)/(b/d)$ or $(a \times d)/(b \times c)$.

Patients	Adverse Event (Case)	No Adverse Event (Control)
Exposed	680	300
Not exposed	125	550

$$
\begin{aligned}
OR &= (680/125)/(300/550); \\
&= 5.44/0.545 \\
&= 9.98
\end{aligned}
$$

(D) How accurate is the estimated risk? We can assess the accuracy of the assessment by examining the CI. A 95% CI refers to the idea that we can be 95% sure that the real measure of risk lies within the given interval. If the interval is large, the risk assessment is considered less precise, which is usually the result of a smaller sample size. To reduce the scope of a CI, a larger sample size will be required. A CI is also important to determine the statistical significance of the assessment.

An RR of 1 implies that there is no difference in risk between the groups and OR 1 implies that the opportunity for the event of interest in a group is the same as the opportunity to have this event in the other group. When the 95% CI includes 1, the assessment of the risk is considered not to be statistically significant; so we can conclude, with 95% confidence, that there is no difference between the two comparison groups.

When the scope of the CI completely falls below or completely above 1, the evaluation is considered to be statistically significant. If, for example, we calculate an OR of 2.0, with a 95% CI: 0.8–3.0, the following conclusions can be drawn: an increase in the possibilities of a result X is observed; however, this increase is not statistically significant.

Conversely, if we calculate an OR of 2.0, with a 95% CI: 1.20–3.0, we could conclude that an increase in the possibilities of obtaining a result X is observed and that this increase is statistically significant.

In conclusion, when the scope of the 95% CI completely falls below or above 1, the evaluation is considered statistically significant. The "positive" outcome of this study is an OR of 9.98 for women using drug I for breast cancer and the risk of intracranial hemorrhage. The 95% CI for this OR was 4.5–14.2. The lowest level of the interval (4.5) is above l; so we can say that there is a positive relationship between intracranial hemorrhage and drug I for breast cancer indication.

No other relationship was found to be statistically significant for this case. For example, men who used drug I for colon cancer appeared to have a lower risk of intracranial hemorrhage (OR: 0.6; IC 95% of 0.20–2.00); however, the interpretation of this in a clinical setting is unclear and unlikely. The 2.00

suggests that we cannot exclude men exposed to drug I from presenting a high risk of intracranial hemorrhage. However, the IC includes 1, which means the assessment of the risk is not considered to be statistically significant.

(E) What is the magnitude of the risk (i.e., its clinical importance)? Even a very high RR or OR does not mean that this relationship is necessarily clinically significant. These measures do not measure current exposure frequency, the rate of recurrence of the problem, or the severity of the problem.

We can assess the magnitude of the risk by using the number of patients needed to treat as a measure (number needed to treat [NNT]).

The NNT is the number of patients you need to treat to prevent an additional bad outcome (death, hemorrhage, etc.). For example, if a drug has an NNT of 3, it means you have to treat three people with the drug to prevent one additional bad outcome.

To calculate the NNT, you need to know the absolute risk reduction (ARR); the NNT is the inverse of the ARR: **NNT = 1/ARR** while ARR = CER (control event rate)—EER (experimental event rate). Then we calculate the harmful effect (number needed to harm [NNH]).

The **NNH** is an epidemiological measure that indicates the average number of patients needed to be exposed to a risk factor over a specific period of time to cause harm in an average of one patient who would not otherwise have been harmed. It is defined as the inverse of the attributable risk.

Intuitively, the lower the number needed to harm, the worse the risk factor is. NNH is similar to NNT, where NNT usually refers to a therapeutic intervention and NNH to a detrimental effect or risk factor. NNH is computed with respect to "exposure" and "nonexposure" and can be determined for raw data or for data corrected for confounders.

A defined end point has to be specified. If the probability *exposure* and *nonexposure* of this end point are known, then the NNH is computed as 1/(*exposure-nonexposure*). This quantity can also be interpreted as the inverse of attributable risk or 1/AR.

The NNH is an important measure in evidence-based medicine and helps physicians decide whether it is prudent to proceed with a particular treatment, which may expose the patient to harm while providing therapeutic benefits. If a clinical end point is devastating enough without the drug (e.g., death, hemorrhage), drugs with a low NNH may still be indicated in particular situations if the NNT (the converse for side effects or the drug's benefit) is less than the NNH.

However, there are several important problems with the NNH, involving bias and lack of reliable CIs, as well as difficulties in excluding the possibility of finding no difference between two treatments or groups. In the present study, the magnitude of the risk has been estimated as 1 (one) woman in 1857, which can undergo an intracranial hemorrhage while taking drug I. The annual frequency of intracranial hemorrhage documented in the medical literature is 0.6 per million per day for people of 45–70 years. This is, however, an estimate based on the calculated OR and may appear clinically important considering that thousands of patients around the world use drug I each year.

Supplementary Information.

Comment # 1 At this point, it is important to understand that, as a general rule, a case-control study cannot be used to calculate the ARR because it is impossible to calculate the impact that can only be calculated in cohort studies or RCT.

When the prevalence of an event is very low, the OR is very close to the RR. In the situation, where the prevalence is low, you should use an equation in which we use the OR to get an approximation of the NNH using two values, either the OR calculated, which is in this case of 9.98 and the expected event rates in patients (expected of patients [PEER event rate]).

According to the literature, the frequency of exposure is 0.6 per million a day for people 45–70 years.

For more information on this equation, please see the following link of the "Center for Evidence-Based Medicine": http://www.cebm.net/number-needed-to-treat-nnt/.

The equation is as follows:

$$\begin{aligned} \text{RIP} &= [(\text{PEER} * [\text{OR} - 1]) + 1]/[\text{PEER} * (\text{OR} - 1) * (1 - \text{PEER})] \\ &= [(0.00006 * [9.98 - 1]) + 1]/[0.00006 * (9.98 - 1) * (1 - 0.00006)] \\ &= [0.00006 * 8.98 + 1]/[0.00006 * 8.98 * 0.99994] \\ &= 10{,}005{,}388/0.0005387677 \\ &= 1857 \text{ people} \end{aligned}$$

For every 1857 patients treated, one (1) patient will have an intracranial hemorrhage.

According to the Council for International Organizations of Medical Sciences (CIOMS) standards, a frequency between ≥1/10,000 and <1/1000 is considered rare (http://www.cioms.ch/).

(F) Should the clinical practice be modified following the results of this study? To answer this question, consider the strength of the association and the model of the study. With a solid study model, i.e., with a well-built RCT, a minimal increase in risk may represent a real harmful effect. On the other hand, should we give a much greater increase in risk to consider a real harmful effect when using a less-extensive study model, such as cohorts and case-control studies?

A small increase in risk in these studies may be the result of subtle flaws in the study model. It must also consider the magnitude of the risk discussed above. Even after having scrutinized all aspects of the study designs, the question of the change in clinical practice can be a difficult question. One must also consider what will be the consequences of a reduction or the elimination of exposure.

Considering the seriousness of this adverse event, specific instructions should also be provided to the health-care providers via the PM to help the identification of patients at risk. These include patients with a history of high blood pressure or a history of arteriovenous malformation, tumors or aneurysm in the brain, family history of intracranial hemorrhage exposure to the anti-inflammatory drugs, anticoagulants, and others.

Specific instructions concerning the treatment of patients with intracranial hemorrhage should also be provided including stopping drug I in the presence of this adverse drug reaction.

Question #3 In our example, there was a high rate of association (OR of 9.98) with the use of this study design, which is sensitive to confounding factors and biases. What regulatory measures, among the following, should be put in place to minimize the risk of intracranial hemorrhage?

(A) Withdraw drug I from the market for only breast cancer indication.
(B) Remove drug I from the market for the indication of colon cancer.
(C) Remove any anti-VEGF from the market for breast cancer indication.
(D) Keep drug I on the market for indications of breast and colon cancer by adding specific safety instructions to the PM, concerning the risk of intracranial bleeding and breast cancer.

Answer: D.

Although there is a strong association (OR of 9.98) between drug I and the intracranial bleeding in women with breast cancer, based on the NNH, it appears that the frequency of this event is rare according to the definition by CIOMS. Based on these results, we can estimate that the benefit/risk ratio remains positive. Thus, it seems unreasonable to recommend the withdrawal of the drug I from the market for breast cancer indication. It is also unreasonable to recommend the withdrawal of the drug I from the market for the indication of colon cancer. Drug I for the treatment of colon cancer is still widely used and has proved its effectiveness in these patients.

Because the information provided does not change significantly the benefit/risk ratio, this indication should not be removed. Even if the drug I has the same molecular entity in the case of the two indications, the doses and the people who use the drug differ, which explains the gap in risk.

Removing all anti-VEGF available on the market for breast cancer indication is not acceptable either. However, these results generate a signal that must be analyzed for other products of the same class on the market, to determine if this risk is associated with the drug I only. If this analysis can also detect a risk of intracranial bleeding for patients with breast cancer, to the other products in the same class, safety measures must be established concerning the indication for breast cancer, including a modification of the standard labeling (PM) for all anti-VEGF, letters to health-care providers and patients.

Therefore, the best answer is to keep drug I on the market for the indication of breast cancer by adding specific safety information related to the risk of intracranial hemorrhage in the PM of this product.

Considering the seriousness of this adverse event, specific instructions should also be provided to help the health-care providers dealing with the identification of at-risk patients, including patients with a history of high blood pressure, a history of arterial–venous malformation, tumors or aneurysm in the brain, a history of intracranial hemorrhage, exposure to antiinflammatory nonsteroidal drugs, anticoagulants, and others.

Specific instructions concerning the treatment of patients with intracranial hemorrhage should also be provided, including discontinuing drug I in the presence of this adverse effect.

4.7 CASE REPORT # 7

4.7.1 Assessment and Management of Serious Adverse Drug Reactions

A 42-year-old woman diagnosed with nephrogenic anemia began a treatment with drug J, a stimulating erythropoietin agent for the treatment of anemia due to chronic renal failure diagnosed a few years ago. The patient received drug J at a dose of 5000 IU intravenously, twice a week. The medical history includes type 1 diabetes mellitus with chronic renal failure on hemodialysis and anemia, secondary to her kidney failure. No concomitant medication is reported.

About 5 months after the start of her treatment with drug J, the patient presented a decline in her hemoglobin to 49 g/L and became dependent on blood transfusions with a reticulocyte count of 36 (N: 10–100). The complete blood count reads: absolute polymorphonuclear eosinophils count of 0.3 (N: 0.0–0.5), absolute lymphocyte count was 1.6 (N: 0.5–3.5), absolute monocyte count was 0.6 (N: 0.2–0.9), absolute neutrophil count was 5.9 (N: 1.5–8), the basophil numeration was 0.1 (N: 0.0–0.1), hematocrit was 0:22 (N: 0:38–0.50), hemoglobin was 69 (N: 130–170), the average corpuscular volume was 28.1 (N: 27–33), the average corpuscular hemoglobin concentration was 332 g/L (N: 320–360), the mean corpuscular volume was 86 (N: 80–97), the mean platelet volume was 8.2 (N: 7–11.5), blood platelet count were 375 (N: 140–400), the number of red blood cells was 2.45 (N: 4.10–5.60), the distribution of red blood cells was 19.4 (N: 12–15), and the number of white blood cells was 8.1 (N: 4–11). Examination of the bone marrow was normocellular but it was made up of 0.4% of mature erythroblasts.

Question #1 Based on the information presented above, what would be your main diagnosis?

(A) Aplastic anemia.
(B) Diamond–Blackfan anemia.

(C) Pure red cell aplasia (PRCA) secondary to treatment with drug J.
(D) Anemia resulting from her underlying diseases.

Answer: C.

(A) Aplastic anemia. Aplastic anemia is the result of damage to the bone marrow and stem cells. This condition causes a deficiency of the three types of blood cells (pancytopenia): red blood cells (anemia), white blood cells (leukopenia), and platelets (thrombocytopenia).

Aplastic refers to the inability of stem cells to generate mature blood cells. It is more common among teens and people in their 20s, but it is also common among the elderly. It can be caused by exposure to chemicals, drugs, radiation, infection, a disease of the immune system, and heredity. In more than half of the cases, the cause is unknown. The definitive diagnosis is confirmed by a biopsy of the bone marrow.

The normal bone marrow contains 30%–70% of stem cells, but in the case of aplastic anemia, these cells are often missing or replaced by fat. Therefore, considering the information presented above, including the absence of a deficit in platelets and white blood cells, aplastic anemia is unlikely.

(B) Diamond–Blackfan anemia. Diamond–Blackfan anemia, also called hereditary PRCA, is a congenital erythroid aplasia present in childhood. This type of anemia presents with a low number of red blood cells (anemia). The rest of the blood is normal including platelets and white blood cells. Therefore, given this patient's medical history, she does not have Diamond–Blackfan anemia. We know that she has anemia, secondary to her kidney failure that started a few years ago, long after childhood. Therefore, this diagnosis is unlikely.

(C) PRCA secondary to treatment with drug J. PRCA is a rare condition that interferes with the formation of erythrocytes (red blood cells). The erythroblasts are almost absent in the bone marrow; however, the production of white blood cells and platelets is normal. These features include severe anemia, fewer than 1% reticulocytes count, and the presence of less than 0.5% of mature erythroblasts in the bone marrow. Examination of the bone marrow is usually normocellular as observed in our patient.

(D) Anemia resulting from her underlying diseases. Anemia is common among people suffering from kidney disease. Healthy kidneys produce a hormone called erythropoietin, which stimulates the bone marrow to produce the appropriate number of red blood cells necessary to transport oxygen to vital organs. Sick kidneys, however, do not produce enough erythropoietin. Thus, the bone marrow produces fewer red blood cells. Other common causes of anemia include loss of blood resulting from hemodialysis and low iron and folic acid levels.

These nutrients, which come from food, help red blood cells to produce hemoglobin, the main protein conveyor of oxygen. A review of the antibody directed against erythropoietin has been requested and proved to be positive, confirming the diagnosis of PRCA associated with taking drug J. Therefore, the best answer is C.

Question #2: Which would be your causality conclusion, if you use the Naranjo algorithm to assess the causal link between this type of anemia and the drug J?

(A) Certain >9;
(B) Probable 5−8;
(C) Possible 1−4;
(D) Unlikely 0.

Answer: C.

According to the Naranjo algorithm, the appearance of this PRCA is possibly related to drug J of the study, with a score of +4. A score of +4 was obtained as follows: there are previous conclusive reports concerning this reaction with the use of drug J [+1], a temporal relationship exists because the adverse effect appeared after the introduction of drug J [+2], and finally, if we refer to the laboratory findings provided in this case report, the presence of PRCA was confirmed by objective evidence [+1]. Therefore, the final score is +4 (possibly related).

Please notice that this assessment should be interpreted with caution, given that no concomitant medication has been listed that could serve as an alternative explanation. The Naranjo score could then be reduced to +2. Despite this possibility, the assessment of this case still would indicate that the event is possibly related to the use of drug J.

Please also note that PRCA was associated with antibodies and has already been reported for months and even years after treatment with other erythropoietin-stimulating agents. Therefore, it is reasonable to suspect drug J as being possibly related to the event of PRCA, which is consistent with the known safety profile of other erythropoietin-stimulating agents.

Question #3: What would you require to make sure that we get an accurate benefit/risk ratio to determine the relationship between drug J and the PRCA event?

(A) A full assessment of similar cases from the databases of clinical trials of the company.
(B) An epidemiological analysis and data from the medical literature.
(C) An assessment of cases of PRCA associated with drug J from the pre- and postapproval activities including the data from Canadian Vigilance and WHO databases.
(D) All of the above.

Answer: D.

Drug J is an erythropoietin-stimulating agent recently authorized for the treatment of nephrogenic anemia by stimulating the action of erythropoietin. PRCA is a known adverse effect associated with several agents of the same class that stimulate erythropoietin. There is preclinical evidence of the relationship between drug J and PRCA.

The effects of intravenous administration of drug J on PRCA have been assessed in rabbits, and this effect was proportional to the doses administered. Therefore, it is possible that the treatment of human patients with drug J is also associated with this adverse effect.

An evaluation of data from clinical trials, epidemiological studies, data from the medical literature, and spontaneous reports from postapproval setting activities have shown a low frequency (<1%) of PRCA in patients receiving drug J. This assessment reveals 50 other cases of PRCA in patients treated with drug J. Even if we find confounding factors associated with this causality assessment, a potential cause and effect relationship cannot be excluded.

Considering that PRCA cases have been reported in clinical context and in postapproval marketing setting and given the seriousness of the event, risk mitigation activities will have to be put in place to ensure the safety of participants in clinical trials and patients in real life, even if the incidence of this adverse effect is low. The goal is to ensure that benefit/risk ratio for drug J remains favorable throughout its life cycle.

Question #4: How you would require that the risk is communicated to ensure the safety of participants in clinical trials and the safety of patients in real life?

(A) Update the IB.
(B) Update the research protocol.
(C) Update the consent form.
(D) Update the PM.
(E) Issue letters to health-care providers and communications to the public.
(F) All of the above.

Answer: F.

Because drug J is still used in clinical trials, updates of the IB, research protocol, and consent form should be made to ensure that researchers and participants in these clinical trials are well informed of this risk.

Because drug J is a health product recently approved, this information should be updated in the PM and should include instructions to health-care providers on how to prevent, identify, and treat this adverse effect. Specific instructions should also be provided regarding the final interruption/stop of this medication when in presence of this adverse drug reaction.

Because drug J is an erythropoietin-stimulating agent and the above risk is a known risk for products of the same class, you should ensure that the labeling of drug J and other drugs of the same class are comparable to each other.

Finally, because PRCA is a serious medical event, this information should be communicated to health-care providers and the public to inform them of the relationship between drug J and this adverse effect.

4.8 CASE REPORT # 8

4.8.1 Disproportionality Analysis in Spontaneous Case Reporting

Drug K is a monoclonal antibody specifically for human B cells used for the treatment of systemic lupus erythematosus. No formal study with drug K has been performed in pregnant women. Currently, it is recommended that drug K should not be used during pregnancy unless it is shown that the potential benefits for the mother justify the potential risk to the fetus.

A search of the Canada Vigilance and WHO databases for spontaneous individual case reports of major congenital malformations reported between January 1, 1995 and September 30, 2016 was made.

This research was conducted to assess for the presence of disproportionality in the spontaneous reporting of the case of major congenital malformations in pregnant women treated with drug K. Events of major congenital malformations associated with drug K were compared to similar events reported in association with other therapies used in the treatment of systemic lupus erythematosus, including biological or antirheumatoid drugs.

The comparison with the standard systemic therapies for systemic lupus erythematosus reduced the possibility of confusion by indication, which may occur in analyses that compare a specific drug to the baseline rate, which includes all drugs.

The analysis involves babies who have been diagnosed with at least a congenital malformation identified at birth or within 12 months after childbirth and are presented by anatomical system or system organ classes (SOC) (see Table 4.1). We take into account the year following childbirth to identify as many congenital defects as possible, given that the diagnosis of congenital malformations can be observed several months after birth. Major congenital malformations have been included and minor malformations have been excluded.

The disproportionality analysis in spontaneous case reporting of major congenital malformations among pregnant women has been evaluated using the proportionality relationship ratio (PRR) and the Bayesian empirical method (Bayes multi-item gamma Poisson shrinker [MGPS]).

When using the PRR method, a signal is detected when the three following conditions are met: (1) at least three cases of the specific adverse event–drug combination have been reported, (2) a PRR of at least 2, and (3) a PRR chi-squared of at least 4.

Based on the empirical method, Bayesian MGPS and the Bayes empirical geometric mean (EBGM) is used to compare the number of events of major congenital malformations associated with drug K to those related to biological and systemic therapies for the treatment of systemic lupus erythematosus.

TABLE 4.1 Analysis of Disproportionality in Spontaneous Reporting of Case Reports of Major Congenital Malformations Associated With Drug K Compared to Other Systemic Therapies Used in the Treatment of Systemic Lupus Erythematosus From the Canada Vigilance and the WHO Databases: From January 1, 1996 to September 30, 2016

Major Congenital Malformations per SOC	Number of Cases	PRR	PRR Chi-Square	EBGM05
Nervous system	35	12	300	3.6
Eyes	2	4	3	0.2
ENT	13	1.1	2.2	1.2
Cardiovascular system	1	1.4	2.5	0.9
Respiratory system	2	1.3	2.4	1.1
Upper digestive tract	8	2.4	6.7	0.8
Lower digestive tract	2	1.4	1.2	0.7
Reproductive system	4	2.9	4.1	1.2
Urinary system	3	1.6	3.2	1.3
Musculoskeletal system	15	6.9	76.3	1.9
Skin	32	3.5	57.7	1.7
Genetic system	1	1.0	0.8	0.9

A potential safety signal based on the Bayesian MGPS method is defined on a threshold of EBGM05 (the lower limit of the one-sided CI of 95% of the EBGM) > 2.

The threshold of signal analysis based on Bayesian MGPS method demonstrates high specificity to detect adverse effects in the safety databases, making it an effective method for assessing the disproportionality reporting of spontaneous case reports of adverse effect.[7,8]

Question #l: Based on the above table, to which of the following major congenital malformations by anatomical system or SOC is drug K a potential related signal?

(A) Nervous system;
(B) Upper digestive tract;
(C) Reproductive system;
(D) Musculoskeletal system.
(E) Skin.

Answer: A.

When we refer to the statistical calculations, outside any clinical context, the term "signal of disproportionality reporting" should be used rather than "signal" to emphasize that the results of this approach may not reflect disproportionality in the reports, which could be affected by many noncausality factors such as the confounding factors, the artifacts, the practice of coding, the underlying diseases, the concomitant medications, or a combination of all these elements.

As well, these results always warrant a more thorough investigation by taking into account the clinical context, because it is known that the systemic lupus erythematosus is associated with a higher frequency of spontaneous abortion, premature delivery, preeclampsia, and early eclampsia or late intrauterine death and poor fetal growth, than the general population.

The systemic lupus erythematosus of the newborn may develop in babies whose mother has systemic lupus erythematosus. These babies may present different disorders, including hydrocephalus.

The disproportionality analysis is not an inferential exercise, that is, the exercise is not intended to draw conclusions on the basis of evidence obtained from a random sample of this population.

The concept of a signal of disproportionality reporting is used to describe a "statistical signal" that originates from an analysis of disproportionality in spontaneous case report reporting.

The underlying principle of this method lies in the fact that the combination drug–event is reported more often than expected in relation to an independent model, based on the frequency of individual case safety reports reported on the drug and the frequency of these reports on a specific adverse event. This statistical relationship implies any sort of causal relationship between the drug and the adverse event.

No golden standard (reference value) currently defines the threshold of disproportionality signals. The PRR is a very sensitive method that can generate a large number of false positive signals, especially when the number of case reports is low. Therefore, the use of the following threshold: (1) at least three cases of the specific adverse event–drug combination being reported, (2) a PRR of at least 2, and (3) PRR chi-squared of at least 4, can reduce the number of false positives. The use of the EBGM05 > 2 threshold is also an approach that provided high specificity to identify signal of disproportionality reporting.

Regarding major congenital malformations reporting by SOC, the nervous system, the upper digestive tract, the reproductive system, the musculoskeletal system and skin have all achieved the number of >3 case reports and a threshold of disproportionality reporting >2 PRR. These systems also reached the PRR Chi-square of at least 4, but only the nervous system has reached the threshold of disproportionality reporting based on the EBGM05 > 2.

Therefore, if we rely on this analysis, we can assume that the major congenital malformations of the nervous system are important potential risks associated with drug K. Please note that the absence of a significant signal of disproportionality reporting does not necessarily exclude the possibility of a link between the health product and the adverse event.

However, because the EBGM05 for the musculoskeletal system is very close to 2, we will certainly continue to follow major congenital malformations related to this system. But for the purposes of this question, A turns out to be the most appropriate answer.

Question #2: Using the analysis of disproportionality reporting, we can properly confirm that there is a link between drug K and major congenital malformations of the nervous system.

True or False.

Answer: False.

The analysis of disproportionality reporting provided a relative frequency of spontaneous reports of adverse events in postapproval marketing phase rather than the incidence of adverse events. The results of such analyses can be used to identify potential safety signals but should not be considered as establishing causal relationships between a drug and a specific adverse event.

There are also limits in the interpretation of data from databases of spontaneous adverse events reports. Spontaneous reporting rates may vary in time and are sensitive to various factors, including the advertising around a specific event in relation to a drug, the lapse of time since the marketing authorization and the sale of a drug (the age of the product), the concerns related to the potential legal aspects of reporting, and other limits.

Differences in the rate of spontaneous reporting for a drug or a specific event may also vary according to the targeted surveillance, the confounding factors (concomitant medication, the patient's medical history, the status of the underlying disease and others), the selective prescription, the motivation of the health-care providers and consumers to report adverse drug-related cases, and the source of the reports (reports from Canadian sources or from foreign sources, from a health-care provider or a consumer). The differences in the rate of spontaneous reports may also vary according to the different signs for a given treatment.

Once a signal is identified, it will be evaluated taking into account (1) the controls of quality as the potential presence of duplicate reports, the completeness of the information contained in these individual reports and coding practices and (2) will take into account medical and clinical assessments regarding adverse events, including the assessment of causality. A signal can be considered a safety signal only after such an assessment is performed.

Question #3: Which of the following approach (es) should be used to properly evaluate a signal?

(A) Identification of potential duplicate reports.
(B) Verification of the data quality.
(C) Getting additional information where necessary.

(D) Verification of the marketing authorization terms.
(E) Verification of any other relevant information.
(F) All of the above.

Answer: F.

As mentioned above, a signal of disproportionality reporting requires a thorough assessment, which takes into account all of the clinical information available concerning the individual case. If necessary, an additional assessment must be made, including, for example, a comparison with other relevant medicinal products.

In general, the use of statistical methods in the detection of signals is useful but requires a thorough knowledge of the available data for a correct interpretation of the results. The steps below provide general guidance on the process of revision of the signal of disproportionality reporting, which relies on medical judgment. These steps should include the following aspects:

(A) Identification of potential duplicate reports. The revision of individual case reports of adverse effects in the analysis of the signal of disproportionality reporting must keep in mind the possibility of having duplicate reports. Although the Canada Vigilance (http://www.hc-sc.gc.ca/dhp-mps/medeff/databasdon/index-eng.php) and WHO (http://www.who.int/medicines/areas/quality_safety/safety_efficacy/advdrugreactions/en/) databases are examined regularly to detect potential duplicates, there may be situations where a report of an individual case is reported more than once and does not initially appear as a potential duplicate report.

(B) Verification of the data quality. Review of the reports of individual cases, in the analysis of the signal of disproportionality reporting, must take into account the completeness of the information provided, the coding practices, and other factors that could influence the quality of the information provided in this individual case.

(C) Gathering of additional information where necessary. Taking into account the information available on the individual case report, it may be necessary to obtain more information from the sender to allow the full assessment of this case. This includes information on the patient himself/herself, his/her underlying diseases, concomitant medication, and others.

(D) Verification of the marketing authorization terms. The PM should be particularly checked to include more information regarding expected as well as known potential drug interactions and known undesirable adverse drug reactions, especially if this product has received an NOC/C.

(E) Verification of any other relevant information. Other information found in the application folder when submitted for obtaining marketing authorization should be taken into account to help in the assessment of the signal of disproportionality reporting, for example, its NDS or SNDS, RMP, PBRER, DSUR, commitments made after marketing authorization, data from postmarketing approval studies, and other relevant information.

Having passed all these stages, no significant causal relationship between drug K and congenital malformations of the nervous system can be made, considering the abovementioned confounding factors such as the underlying disease, concomitant medication, and others. However, it is essential to keep following the evolution of this adverse effect observed with the use of drug K and implement regulatory measures, as required, to minimize this adverse effect.

The change in the labeling of the PM, the communication of new information to health-care providers and to the public, and other measures are relevant to ensure the safety of patients.

Question #4: Based on the above information, at this point, no other precautionary measure is necessary because the regulator and the investigator follow the case closely.

True or False.

Answer: False.

To monitor birth defects in pregnant women exposed to drug K, a registry of pregnant women should be established. Health-care professionals are encouraged to enroll pregnant women in this registry. Similarly, pregnant women who receive drug K are encouraged to register themselves in this registry.

As discussed earlier, a registry is a list of patients who have the same characteristic. This feature can be defined as a disease (disease registry) or a specific exposure to a drug (drug registry). The two types of registry, which differ only on the type of data of interest, can help provide information using a standardized questionnaire, on a prospective basis.

Disease registries: A disease registry can also be used as a database for a case-control study to compare exposure to the drug of the cases identified in the registry to patients-selected controls in the registry with another condition, or to patients from outside the registry.

Exposure registry (drug registry): Certain drug registries address exposures to drugs in specific populations, such as pregnant women as in this case. Other activities of active surveillance may also be adopted, including the sentinel sites, active surveillance protocols, tracking of specific events, or comparative observational studies.

4.9 CASE REPORT # 9

4.9.1 Superiority Trials to Establish Drug Safety

Drug N is an insulin product recently authorized for marketing and is indicated for the treatment of patients with type 1 or type 2 insulin-dependent diabetes mellitus. Therefore, the efficacy and safety of drug N for these indications have already been demonstrated in previous clinical trials. The manufacturer wants to demonstrate that this biological product newly arrived on the market is superior to another insulin of the same class already on the market (drug O), with regard to the risk of specific adverse effects, when used in optimal and comparable conditions. The manufacturer implemented a phase IV study to compare drug N and drug O about the risks of specific adverse effects.

**A phase IV study is a study of an approved indication and is conducted following approval of the sale of a drug by a regulator. These studies are often important to optimize the use of drugs. They may be of any type but must include valid scientific objectives. Among the most common studies, some are related to safety and some seek to confirm usage within the approved indication, such as mortality/morbidity studies and epidemiological studies.*

Question #1: Which type of study would be most recommended to answer this question adequately?

(A) Cohort study.
(B) Case-control study.
(C) Cross-sectional study.
(D) Double-blind randomized controlled trial.
(E) Metaanalysis.
(F) Systematic review of the medical literature.

Answer: D.

(A) Cohort study: As discussed in Case Report # 6, in a cohort study, a population of patients at risk of presenting the disease or an adverse drug reaction in particular is followed in time to check for the appearance of the said disease or adverse drug reaction. Exposure information is collected throughout the follow-up period with each patient and can be compared with nonexposed patients (controls). Given that the exposure in the follow-up population is known, the incidence rate can be calculated. Several adverse drug reactions can also be studied using the same data source with this kind of study.

As for case-control studies, the identification of patients for cohort studies can come from automated databases. In addition, cohort studies can be used to examine safety issues in specific populations (elderly, children, and patients with comorbidity, pregnant or nursing women, and others). Given the purpose of this study, which is to demonstrate that drug N is superior to drug O regarding drug safety, it is best to set up a double-blind RCT that allows for an accurate assessment of drugs N and O. Therefore, A is not the best answer.

(B) Case-control studies. As noted in 1C of Case Report # 6, in a case-control study, cases of disease (or events) are identified. Controls or patients without illness or events of interest are then selected from the population of origin, which has given rise to cases of disease (or events). Controls should be selected to ensure that the prevalence of exposure among the controls represents the prevalence of exposure in the original population.

Case-control studies are used to highlight the factors that may contribute to the onset of a disease or event of interest by comparing subjects that have this disease or event of interest (cases) with subjects who did not have the disease or event of interest, but are similar (controls).

The status of the exposure in the two groups is then compared with the OR, which is an estimate of the RR of disease (or events) in the exposed, compared to the nonexposed. If safety concerns are found in specific populations, the cases and controls can be stratified into target populations (the elderly, children, pregnant women, and others).

Case-control studies are particularly useful when the purpose of the study is to examine whether there is a link between a drug and a rare specific adverse event, as well as to identify the risk of adverse factors. A case-control study could also be put in place to identify and quantify the risks (case-control surveillance).

Therefore, as the objective of the current study is to demonstrate that drug O is superior to drug N concerning their respective safety profile, a case-control study is not the best approach to answer the question asked by the manufacturer.

(C) Cross-sectional studies (surveys). For these studies, data are collected on a population of patients (or a representative sample of patients) at a single point in time (or time interval), regardless of the status of exposure or disease. This type of study is mainly used to collect data from surveys or for environmental analyses (studies of the population rather than individuals).

The major drawback of cross-sectional studies is that the temporal relationship between exposure and adverse event(s) cannot be directly determined. These studies are most useful to study the prevalence of a disease at a specific point in time or to look at trends over time, when the annual (temporal) data can be obtained.

These studies can also be used to examine the raw association between exposure and adverse effects in environmental analyses. Cross-sectional studies are most useful when exposure does not change over time. Therefore C is not the best answer.

(D) Double-blind randomized controlled trial: Where significant risks are identified in preapproval phase, double-blind RCT can be conducted to evaluate the mechanism of action of certain adverse drug reactions in post-approval settings.

In some cases, PK and PD studies can be conducted to determine whether a particular dose of the medication can put patients at increased risk of adverse reactions. Genetic tests can also provide information on groups of patients with an increased risk of adverse effects. In addition, investigation of possible food and drug interactions studies can also be performed, where necessary.

Sometimes, the potential or unintended risks in specific populations could not be identified during clinical trials before marketing approval. These potential or unintended risks may not have been fully quantified due to the small sample size or the exclusion of patient subpopulations from these clinical trials. These people include the elderly, children, or patients with kidney or liver disorders. In addition, children, the elderly, and those suffering from comorbidity may metabolize drugs differently from patients generally included in clinical trials.

Clinical trials could be used to identify and quantify the magnitude of the risk in these populations. RCT that has a primary safety outcome can be an important tool for active surveillance of adverse drug reactions because the randomization of subjects is expected to interpret an association of causality between exposure to the drug and one or more adverse effects. Double-blind means that neither the investigator nor the participants know which health product a patient receives, which eliminates a lot of bias that could invalidate the study. In addition, RCT remains the most rigorous method to compare two treatments. For these last reasons a double-blind RCT is the best approach to answer the question asked by the manufacturer. Therefore D is the best answer.

(E) Metaanalyses. Unlike a direct comparison used in cohort studies, case-control or RCT, the use of indirect comparison studies such as the meta-analysis or systematic reviews of the literature (see F) compare the effects of interventions to each other, based on their performance versus a common comparator.[9,10]

The quantitative results of several similar studies comparing outcomes of an intervention with the same comparator can be combined by means of a metaanalysis to sum up the available evidence from a combined estimate on a variable of interest (metaanalysis in pairs). In addition, different comparisons either from different interventions can be combined in a metaanalysis of the network (also known as joint treatment comparisons or metaanalyses of multiple treatments).[9,10]

A crucial concept in indirect comparisons is to make sure not to break the initial random selection, and in this way, maintain the benefits of the double-blind RCT. For example, if a test compares a drug with a placebo and a second test compares drug B to a placebo, it is wrong to simply compare the absolute efficacy observed with drug A compared to that observed with drug B. Indeed, part of the absolute efficacy can be attributed to the drug, whereas another part of efficacy may also be due to a placebo effect. In addition, differences in the absolute treatment effects may be the result of confounding factors.[11] The basic assumptions underlying the indirect comparisons involve that the results of these tests should be sufficiently homogeneous.

In fixed effects models, it is assumed that the differences between the treatment effects are caused only by the difference in treatment, not by any other confounding factor. In random effects models, differences in the effects of a specific study treatment (beyond the differences attributable to the interventions being compared) are exchangeable and the heterogeneity is constant between different comparisons.[12]

Another hypothesis validating an adjusted indirect comparison is the similarity. This means that patients included must be sufficiently similar so that the relative estimated effect for trials A against C is generalizable to patients in trials B against C and that the relative effect estimated by trials B against C be generalizable to the patients in the trials A against B.[13]

Finally, when direct and indirect evidence is available, an assumption of coherence is necessary to combine direct and indirect estimates quantitatively.[13] The possible causes of divergence (or inconsistency) between direct and indirect evidence include: (1) the elements of chance, (2) the invalidity of indirect comparisons, (3) the presence of bias in face-to-face comparative studies, and (4) clinically significant heterogeneity between trials.[13]

The findings of a metaanalysis are obtained by applying a statistical inference technique, which can be either frequentist or Bayesian.[14] With a frequentist approach, the result of the metaanalysis is a point estimate with a 95% CI. The Bayesian methods involve a formal a priori probability combination distribution (which reflects the a priori belief of the possible values of the pooled treatment effect) with a common distribution probability effect based on data observed to obtain a posteriori probability distribution of the pooled treatment effect.[14]

The probability tells us the extent in which the different values for the parameter of interest are supported by the data. Therefore, the treatment effect a posteriori distribution obtained with the Bayesian approach can be interpreted in terms of probabilities, allowing a more intuitive interpretation of the results.[14]

Although increasingly adopted to compare different treatments effects in many medical fields, the indirect comparisons do not escape the conceptual and technical challenges. As the compared treatments are not directly randomized, the standard metaanalysis only provides observational evidence and has some limitations compared to direct observational studies.[13]

In addition, some inconsistencies can be explained even after elimination of the confounding factors. Indeed, a recent metaepidemiologic study has identified 14% inconsistency between direct and indirect comparisons.[15] Therefore, metaanalyses study is not as effective as a face-to-face study to compare drugs O with N. For these reasons, E is not the best answer.

(F) Systematic review of the medical literature. A systematic review is a thorough, comprehensive, and explicit interview of the medical literature. It usually includes several steps, among which the authors (1) ask questions that can be answered (often the most difficult step), (2) identify one or more databases in which to query, (3) develop an explicit research strategy, (4) select titles, summaries, and texts based on explicit criteria, to make them decide which scientific articles or nonscientific texts should be kept, and (5) summarize the data from these articles in a standardized format.

A systematic review must be distinguished from a metaanalysis, which is a statistical approach to combine data from a systematic review (see E).

Therefore, any metaanalysis should be based on an underlying systematic review, whereas all systematic reviews do not necessarily give place to a metaanalysis.

For more information about systematic literature reviews, see the Cochrane handbook (http://training.cochrane.org/handbook) at the Resources for Readers section. Because a systematic review is also an indirect comparison method, it is not the best approach for the comparison between the drugs N and O. For these reasons again, D remains the best answer.

Supplementary Information.

Comment # 1 The choice of the control group is always a critical decision in the design of a clinical trial. This choice affects the inferences that can be drawn from the study including the ethical acceptability of the trial, the degree to which the bias can be minimized, and the realization and analysis of the study results.

This choice also affects the type of study that can be used and the pace of recruitment, the kind of end result indicators (end points) that can be studied, the scientific credibility, and the acceptability of the results by the regulations authorities and several other features of the study.

The choice of the control group should be considered as part of the standard therapies and bears an impact on the evidence supporting the design and for the study ethical considerations. For more information regarding the choice of the control group, the reader should consult the ICH E10 Guidelines at the Resources for the Readers section.

Question #2: The manufacturer therefore opts for a double-blind RCT comparing drugs N and O because the most important safety variables clinically predefined are known to be associated with the use of these two types of insulin. The manufacturer issued as a hypothesis that drug N is superior to drug O with respect to the risk of common adverse effects known to be associated with insulin.

Among the following statements what should be its comparison objective(s) and why?

(A) Demonstrate that drug N is superior to drug O.
(B) Demonstrate that drug N is equivalent to drug O.
(C) Demonstrate that drug N is noninferior to drug O.
(D) None of the above.
(E) Only the statements A and C are acceptable.

Answer: A.

(A) Demonstrate that drug N is superior to drug O. In a superiority trial, the goal is to show that a new treatment is better than the standard treatment or the comparator. In this case, the manufacturer must demonstrate that drug N is superior to drug O with respect to the risk of adverse drug reactions.

The hypothesis assumes that the difference between the averages of the two groups is zero or negative, that is, it promotes the standard treatment of drug O compared to the alternative hypothesis, which assumes that the new drug (drug N) is preferable. The desirable difference in the treatment effects should be decided on a clinical basis, taking into account the disease characteristic, the proven control therapy, and what can reasonably be expected from this new therapy.

The purpose of a superiority trial implies that researchers are not interested in results that show if new drug (drug N) is equal to or less efficient than the standard treatment with drug O, but to demonstrate that drug N is superior to drug O for the safety variables studied. However, a gap in this type of test is that significant results in the opposite direction must be rejected, despite their potential to be clinically significant.

For more information about the superiority trial design, please consult the EMA Guidelines: Tests of superiority and noninferiority, at the Resources for Readers section or visit the following link: http://www.ema.europa.eu/docs/en_GB/document_library/Scientific_guideline/2009/09/WC500003658.pdf.

According to this Guideline, in a test of good quality, the degree of statistical significance ("*P*" value) indicates the probability that the observed difference—or a larger one—should be caused by chance to assume there was really no difference between treatments. Lower this probability, rending increasingly implausible that there is no difference between the treatments. Once it is admitted that the hypothesis of "no difference" is eliminated, it becomes important to estimate the size of the difference to assess whether the effect is clinically relevant.

It is essential that this CI do not contain a 0 as the possibility of no difference has already been rejected as unreasonable.

Thus, the two following items are generally considered equivalent: (1) the two-sided 95% CI for the difference between means excludes 0; (2) the two means are statistically different at the 5% level ($P < .05$) two sided.

When the meaning is mentioned in practice, specific numerical values of probabilities are generally cited, for example $P = .032$, as this value is more informative than $P < .5$.

This allows judging, specifically, the magnitude of the differences between the null hypothesis and the observed data, rather than on approximations such as 0:05, 0:01 to 0.001. However, CIs must be associated with a given probability limit value and here, the interval of 95% is almost always considered.

When a difference is statistically significant at a more extreme level, for example $P = .002$, the two-sided 95% CI will exclude 0 by a wider margin.

Fig. 4.1 illustrates these points. To get more information about the superiority trials, please consult the EMA Guidelines on the superiority and noninferiority trials, at the Resources for Readers section or visit the following link: http://www.ema.europa.eu/docs/en_GB/document_library/Scientific_guideline/29/09/WC500003658.pdf.

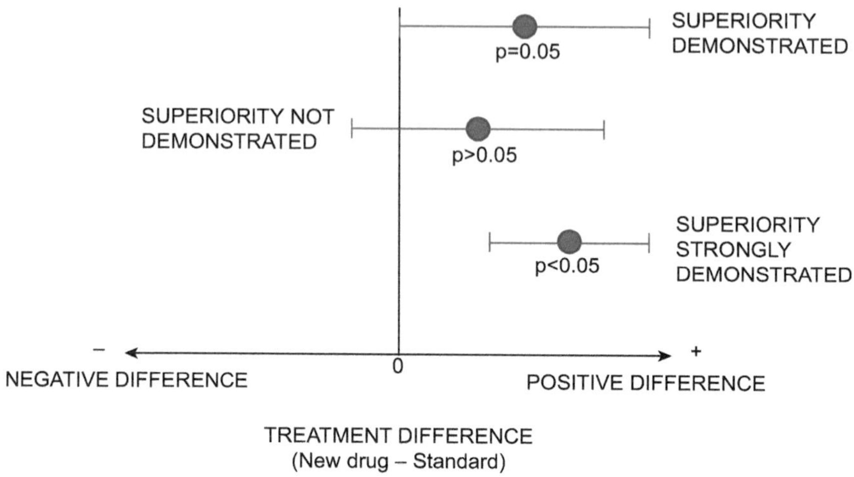

FIGURE 4.1 Demonstrations of superiority based on the level of significance and the confidence interval.

To determine whether the observed difference is indeed relevant is a matter of judgment. Unlike an equivalence or noninferiority trial where the clinical relevance is considered by the prestudy choice of "a clinical equivalence margin (Δ)" (see also B and C), in a superiority trial the clinical relevance requires to consider separate conditions and a statistically significant difference maybe not clinically relevant. The difference taken as the basis of power calculation in a superiority trial cannot be assumed to provide a suitable value.

Note that in Fig. 4.1 and in the rest of this case report, it is assumed that the values to the right of 0 correspond to a better response to the new treatment, whereas the values to the left of 0 indicate that the standard treatment or the comparator is better. Because the objective of this study is to demonstrate that drug N is superior to drug O, A is the better answer.

(B) Demonstrate that drug N is equivalent to drug O. An equivalence trial is designed to confirm the absence of significant difference between two treatments. Because it is basically impossible to prove that two treatments are exactly equivalent, "a clinical equivalence margin (Δ)" must be determined. The assumption is that the difference between the treatments is outside the interval, compared to the alternative hypothesis, which assumes that the differences lie within this range (Δ). This last is selected by setting the important clinically acceptable difference, so that any bigger gap would be important in practice.

If both treatments must be declared equivalent, then the 95% bilateral CI (two sided), which defines the range of plausible differences between two

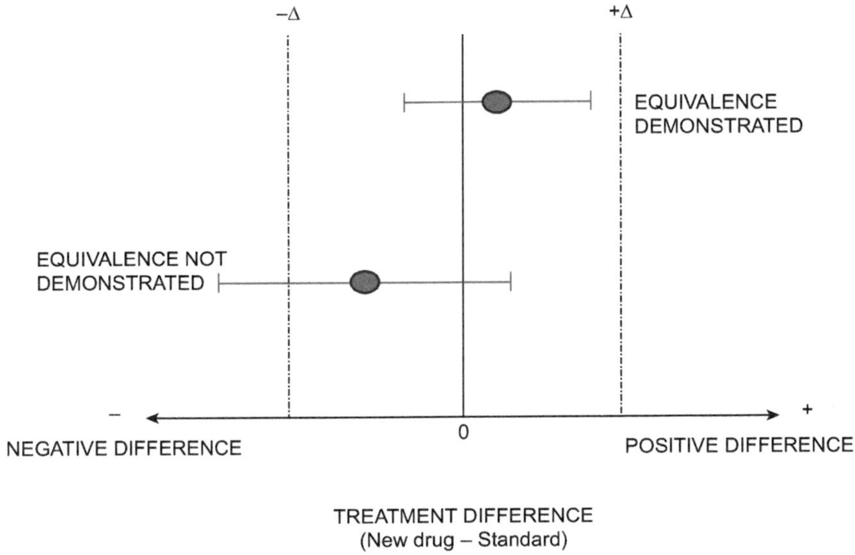

FIGURE 4.2 Demonstrations of equivalence based on the confidence interval.

treatments should be entirely within the range from $-\Delta$ to $+\Delta$ (see Fig. 4.2). These equivalency tests are often performed when a BBD or a generic enters the market. Here considering that drug N is not a BBD of drug O, B is not the best answer. For more information, please consult the EMA Guidelines at the Resources for Readers section or visit the following link: http://www.ema.europa.eu/docs/en_GB/document_library/Scientific_guideline/2009/09/WC500003658.pdf.

(C) Demonstrate that drug N is noninferior to drug O. In studies of drug development, noninferiority trials are more frequent than the equivalence trial. These trials aim at showing that a new treatment is not worse than an existing treatment: either it can be more effective and safer or it can have a similar effect. Here again, a CI approach is the easiest way to do the analysis, but in this case, we are interested only in a possible one-direction difference.

The null hypothesis is that the new drug is not as good as the standard treatment up to a certain point, whereas the alternative hypothesis states that the superiority of the standard drug does not exceed this interval. That is why the 95% confidence bilateral interval (two sided) must be completely to the right of the $-\Delta$ value (see Fig. 4.3).

However, given that noninferiority trials do not include a true negative control group, the results of these tests are analyzed carefully and are not

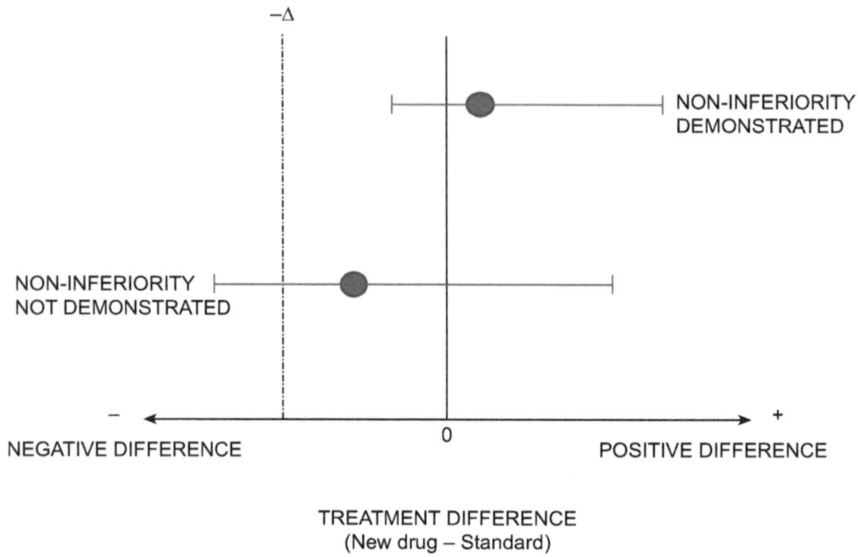

FIGURE 4.3 Demonstrations of noninferiority based on the confidence interval.

generally accepted as being as strong as those obtained during a superiority trial. In the current case the objective is to demonstrate that drug N is superior to drug O. Therefore A is the best answer.

4.10 CASE REPORT # 10

4.10.1 Important Safety Issues to Consider in the Development of a New Drug

P is a human immunoglobulin of high affinity directed against the receptors of the human epidermal growth factor # 3 (HER-3), which is expressed in Chinese hamster ovarian cells (CHO). HER-3 receptor is a transmembrane glycoprotein, which is expressed in many normal tissues and in a variety of solid tumors, including lung cancer, breast cancer, colon cancer, ovarian cancer, and others. Higher levels of HER-3 receptors have been associated with a negative clinical prognosis, including a decrease in survival in several types of solid tumors.

Therefore, it is logical to believe that an antibody that blocks the specific signal of this HER-3 transmembrane receptor could have significant clinical effects.

The mechanism of action of drug P is not new and is similar to other products acting on similar family receptors already available on the market.

Drug P is in development and is used in clinical studies for the indications of lung cancer and in other advanced solid tumors with positive HER-3 receptors named metastatic breast cancer.

Question 1. Which of the following safety concerns should you suspect with this product?

(A) A potential effect on heart function.

(B) A potential effect on lung function.

(C) A potential effect on liver function.

(D) A potential effect on the QT/QTc interval.

(E) A potential effect on immunogenicity.

(F) Possible reactions of hypersensitivity/infusion related.

(G) Other potential safety issues based on the findings from products of the same class.

(H) All of the above concerns are true.

Answer: H.

(A) A potential effect on heart function. Cardiac toxicity was observed with other products acting on HER-receptors family. The nonclinical and clinical data with drug P do not support an effect of this drug on heart function.

As well, the acquisition (MUGA) scans showed no significant reduction in the ejection fraction in presence of drug P suggesting, to date, an absence on ventricular dysfunction or congestive heart failure in patients taking drug P.

Therefore, this potential effect and the other effect mentioned here require to be followed with a lot of rigor throughout the development and following commercialization of drug P if this product is authorized for marketing (i.e., throughout the life cycle of drug P). This demonstrates the importance of looking at other products of the same class to make a complete assessment of the current product.

(B) A potential effect on lung function. Data from other products in the HER family of receptors have identified an effect on the respiratory system as a safety concern for this class of products. The information provided by the development program of drug P to date does not support a toxic effect of drug P on lung function. Also note that pulmonary toxicity can also occur as a result of a drug infusion–related reaction (see also F).

(C) A potential effect on liver function. Liver toxicity has been identified with another product from the HER-receptor family. Adverse effects in liver function have been reported with drug P mainly in studies where it has been used in combination with another drug of the same class.

However, information from drug P development program does not support an effect of this drug on the liver function. It is important to remember that drug hepatotoxicity is one of the most frequent reasons to refuse marketing or at least restrict the use of new drugs in development. Hepatotoxicity is also the main reason to withdraw a marketing authorization already granted to a product.

Therefore, drug hepatotoxicity is a major concern during the development phase and during the postapproval phase of a health product (i.e., throughout the life cycle of a product).

To facilitate the work of developers, Health Canada provides them with Guidelines regarding the assessment of hepatotoxicity during the premarketing development of health products with the aim of exposing the elements to be considered so that they meet the requirements and find how to avoid and manage the risks of hepatotoxicity. This includes the detection, assessment, and mitigation of adverse reactions related to hepatotoxicity caused by health products use by humans, alone or in combination with other health products, prior to marketing approval.

The reader is invited to browse this Guideline that can be found at Resource for Readers section for more information on premarket evaluation of hepatotoxicity of health products.

(D) A potential effect on the QT/QTc interval. The effect of drug P on the QT/QTc interval has been studied by ECG data gathered from about 350 subjects. The ECG data analysis indicates that the probability that drug P could have a significant impact on the QT interval and the QT interval corrected (QTc), heart rate, is seen as being very low.

As you know, because of its inverse relationship with the heart rate, the measurement of QT interval is routinely transformed by using formulas for heart rate correction in a variable called QT interval corrected, which is independent of the heart rate. Thus, an excessive prolongation of the QT/QTc interval creates an electrophysiologic environment for the occurrence of a twist of spikes, a polymorphic ventricular tachyarrhythmia that can result in syncope or evolve into a ventricular fibrillation and sudden cardiac death. To facilitate the work of developers, Health Canada provides Guidelines for the analysis and review of the data on the QT/QTc interval that can be used as a guide for a good understanding of this interval and the response required based on the data on this interval.

This document should be used in combination with the ICH E14 Guidelines on the clinical assessment of the risk of QT/QTc interval prolongation and pro-arrythmics effects of non-antiarrhythmic drugs. All the clinical information related to drug P and its impact on QT/QTc intervals should be included in the PM for this product. This Guidelines is available at the Resources for Readers section.

(E) A potential effect on immunogenicity. As biological drugs are produced or extracted from living organisms, these products are considered by the human body as foreign bodies and therefore promote the appearance of an acute and/or chronic immune response. However, in clinical studies with drug P, the impact of antihuman antibodies has been very low and no neutralizing antibodies were found in the treated group.

(F) Possible reactions of hypersensitivity/infusion-related reactions. As with all biological products, administration of drug P causes a potential risk of hypersensitivity reactions or infusion-related reactions (see also B because pulmonary toxicity may also be an infusion-related reaction). No increased risk of infusion-related reactions and hypersensitivity reactions with drug P has been confirmed in previous studies.

Nevertheless, the risk of hypersensitivity is important and will set up a contraindication in the presence of hypersensitivity to drug P, to proteins of the CHO cells, or to any ingredient of the product. To comply with the recommendations on the PM see the Guidelines that can be found at the Resources for Readers section.

(G) Other potential safety issues based on the findings from a product of the same class. Additional potential risks based on the findings from products of the same class should be rigorously evaluated and could be signals to be followed, not only in premarket but also in postmarketing settings (i.e., throughout the life cycle of drug P), if the product is authorized for marketing.

Question 2. Which of the following parameters for additional safety should you also consider to get a better safety profile in the development of drug P?

(A) The effects on the kidney and liver function.

(B) Drug interactions.

(C) The results of laboratory tests.

(D) The use of drug P during pregnancy and lactation.

(E) The experience with using drug P in the long term.

(F) The considerations regarding medication errors overdose and drug abuse.

(G) The lack of efficacy of drug P

(H) The experience with the use of drug P in special populations.

(I) All the abovementioned parameters are true.

Answer: I.

(A) The effects on kidney and liver function. As the dose of the health product may need to be adjusted in patients with renal or hepatic failure or impairment, and thus have an impact on the safety profile of drug P, it is essential to evaluate these functions in specific PK studies.

In the case presented here, the effects of kidney and liver failure and impairments on the PK parameters of drug P were evaluated in a specific PK study. The analysis of these parameters does not suggest any apparent effect of hepatic or renal failure or impairment in using drug P.

In addition, drug P has not demonstrated any modifications in any PK parameters when exposed to concomitant administration of other drugs. This indicates that no adjustment in the dosage of drug P is necessary in presence of the kidney or hepatic failure or impairments.

(B) Drug interactions. It is essential to obtain information about drug interactions because it can influence the needs of drug P. In fact, it can increase or decrease the dose needed to get the desired effect with this drug. In addition, the presence of a drug interaction can exacerbate a specific adverse effect.

Regarding drug P, no signs or symptoms has been observed suggesting a clinically significant drug interaction with concurrent health products used in clinical studies. However, this aspect of the safety profile should be followed in postapproval epidemiological studies if the product is authorized. In addition to the drug–drug interaction, it is necessary to check the drug–food interactions and medicinal drug–herb interactions. These interactions also need to be documented in the PM if drug P receives marketing authorization.

(C) The results of laboratory tests that are affected by the presence of the drug can change the precision of the results of the test or methods used and thus indirectly have an impact on the safety profile of drug P. For the case discussed here, no clinically significant trend has been identified after a review of adverse reactions, during the analysis of laboratory test results, vital signs, ECG, and others, in studies conducted with Drug P.

(D) The use of drug P during pregnancy and lactation. Because an embryo–fetal toxicity was identified in the postmarket setting with other products acting on HER receptors family, it is essential to determine if drug P entails similar risks. With drug P, there has been no adverse human experience during pregnancy and lactation.

However, if the product is authorized for marketing, special precautions must be taken to minimize the risk of embryo–fetal toxicity in pregnant women treated with drug P. These precautions will have to be clearly stated in the PM following the recommendations of the PM guidelines.

When a drug is absorbed systemically, information on excretion in breast milk and its effects on the infant must be documented. Predictable adverse reactions in infants should be mentioned in the PM and measures should be recommended to avoid high exposure in infants. The potential for serious or oncogenic adverse effects must be clearly identified. In the absence of data from clinical studies in lactating women, relevant data from studies carried out in animals must be mentioned in the PM.

In addition, a statement should be clearly mentioned in the PM, indicating that precautions should be taken in these patients if no information is available on whether or not drug P is excreted in breast milk. The choice of giving drug P in pregnant or lactating women should be based on the benefits for the mother and on the risks for the child. The benefits should always outweigh the risks.

(E) The experience with using drug P in the long term. In clinical studies in general, there is often a lack of information on the effects in the long-term use of a drug that will most possibly be seen with epidemiological studies in postapproval marketing (i.e., throughout the product life cycle). This information in the long-term use of drug P is likely to change its benefit/risk ratio. Long-term security data monitoring of drug P have been collected in several clinical studies.

Currently, no specific security concern has been raised after more than 124 weeks of processing, but data should be followed throughout the development of this product and after the marketing authorization, if drug P is authorized for marketing, to ensure that the benefit/risk ratio remains favorable at long term for more than 2 years.

(F) The considerations regarding medication errors overdose and drug abuse. Because drug P is in clinical development, there has been no experience with this health product so far showing clinically significant medication errors, overdose, or drug abuse in humans. Once again, in the context of clinical trials, it is difficult to verify these aspects of the safety profile of drug P. This may be evaluated in postapproval setting if drug P is authorized. Of course, if appropriate, instructions should be mentioned in the PM to prevent these considerations and to determine how to treat them.

(G) Lack of efficacy of drug P. Data indicating a lack of efficacy may reflect a significant risk for participants in clinical trials and should be considered with a lot of rigor. During the development program, there is no evidence suggesting a lack of efficacy of drug P. In addition, no information is known to date suggesting a lack of efficacy on any high-risk patient populations. Of course, a potential lack of efficacy will be followed throughout the development of drug P.

(H) Experience with the use of drug P in special populations. It is very difficult in the context of clinical trials to obtain information in some populations. However, it may be assessed in postapproval settings. Thus, in the case discussed here, drug P was not formally studied in subjects below 18 years old or in the elderly.

However, according to the ongoing clinical development program, 154 elderly people >65 years are included in these studies. No safety finding has been identified in data from the elderly >65 years so far. Nevertheless, this population should be followed throughout the development of drug P.

Other considerations: In the case presented here, during the development program of drug P, it is important to question for the presence of problems related to treatment adherence and other manufacturing considerations that could affect the safety of patients participating in these clinical studies. In addition, it is also important to determine for any new information concerning the safety of drug P identified from the analysis of nonclinical data, the medical literature pharmacoepidemiological studies or data from other similar products in the same class.

4.11 CASE REPORT # 11

4.11.1 How to Evaluate an Article Discussing Treatment or Prevention Strategies

As a student in various fields, professor, or health-care provider when you have to evaluate an article discussing the treatment or prevention strategies for specific diseases, what are the questions you should ask to yourself before deciding if the article is useful in making a decision for your clinical practice or for your learning?

Question # 1: Among the following, which are the elements that may help you decide whether or not the study is valid?

(A) Randomization procedure;
(B) Treatment groups similar to the control group except for the interventions;
(C) Blinding procedure;
(D) Intention to treat analysis:
(E) Excessive loss to follow-up;
(F) All of the above are correct.

Answer: F.

(A) Randomization procedure: The randomization procedure certainly improves your study design by assuring (most of the time) that both known and unknown factors that could impact the outcome of the study are equally distributed. Non-randomized studies very often may lead to the wrong conclusion that a treatment has a beneficial effect when it is not true. For example, a study of Trintellix (an antidepressant) on smoking cessation may help select for individuals already motivated to stop smoking unless treatment and control groups are randomized.

(B) Treatment groups similar to the control group except for the interventions: This is a very important element that could greatly impact the validity of the study and for that you should take a look at the subjects section but most of the time you look for tables showing baseline patient characteristics other than the intervention. Significant differences between the two groups (even if by chance) will make it very difficult to attribute the results to the study intervention. For example, some trials of new therapies for cancer allow steroid use, which can significantly alter the laboratory values and alter the quality of life questionnaires (steroids are also pain killers).

(C) Blinding Procedure: The expectations of patients or health-care providers can influence the outcomes if the study is not blinded (introduce selection bias and others). If patient, health-care providers, or both were blinded, then those evaluating outcomes should not be aware of the assigned treatment groups.

(D) Intention to treat analysis: This is also an important concept in clinical research. In an intention to treat analysis patients remain in the original group to which they were randomized regardless of what treatment they received. This will prevent unknown factors that can influence treatment from affecting the reported outcome. For example, if patients left the study group for the control group because of worsening clinical status in a randomized controlled trial of a new therapy for congestive heart failure, the study may have a positive outcome not because the new therapy was effective but because the patients with worse disease left the control group.

(E) Excessive loss to follow-up: This is also an important concept where patients who are lost to follow-up tend to have different outcomes than patients who complete a study. This can bias a study either for or against a treatment. You can decide if there was excessive loss to follow-up by reassessing the conclusions. Assume that all lost subjects had a negative outcome in a positive study or that they had a positive outcome in a negative study. If the conclusions change, this was due to an excessive loss to follow-up.

Question # 2: Among the following items, which are the elements that may help you decide whether or not the results are valid or relevant?

(A) ARR;
(B) RR;
(C) Relative risk reduction (RRR);
(D) NNT;
(E) CI and *P*-value;
(F) All of the above are correct.

Answer: F.

(A) ARR: The ARR is the absolute difference between the proportion who suffered an event in the control group and the proportion who presented the same adverse event in the treatment group. If X = the proportion of patients presenting a specific adverse event in the control group such as myocardial infarction and Y = the proportion of patients in the treatment group who had the same event, then ARR = X − Y.

(B) RR: The RR is the ratio of events among patients that receive the treatment to the events in control patients. RR = Y/X (see Chapter 3).

(C) RRR: The RRR is the most common way to report treatment differences. It is the percentage in which a treatment reduces risk of an event relative to the risk in the control patients. RRR = [1 − (Y/X)] × 100%. If the risk of myocardial infarction in a population receiving a new treatment is 10% and the risk of myocardial infarction in the control population is 20%, then the new treatment reduces the risk of myocardial infarction by 50% compared with the baseline risk (RRR = 50%).

(D) NNT: The NNT helps to determine if the benefits of a therapy are worth the costs and potential harm of the therapy. NNT can serve as a more practical way of thinking about results. NNT = 1/ARR. An equivalent RRR but quite different NNT is obtained from the following examples. Consider that the risk of myocardial infarction for the two different treatment populations is 25% and 0.5% compared with baseline risks of 50% and 1%, respectively. The RRR for either treatment is 50%, but the NNT for the first treatment is 4 (4 patients would need to be treated to prevent one myocardial infarction) and the NNT for the second treatment is 200 (200 patients would need to be treated to prevent one myocardial infarction). Although the RRR is equal, the first treatment would have a larger influence on your clinical practice especially if treatment is costly or not well tolerated.

(E) CI and *P*-value: CIs define the range in which the true effect lies. We arbitrarily use 95% CIs to define statistical significance. The true result will lay beyond the CIs 5% of the time (2.5% above the upper boundary and 2.5% below the lower boundary of the 95% CI). The *P*-value gives the probability that the result is due to chance alone. *P*-values less than .05 are considered statistically significant.

Question # 3: True or False. After analyzing all the elements above, we should be able to answer whether or not the results help in taking care of your patients.

Answer: True.

After examining the results you should be able to decide whether or not the results apply to your patients. For that you need to ask whether your patient would be included in the study by looking at the inclusion and exclusion criteria as well as the features of reported subgroups. Also, you should look to see if the outcome studied is clinically relevant or has no clinical significance. You should also ask yourself whether the treatment adversely affects other outcomes not studied in the trial. You should perform a benefit/risk ratio assessment and the benefits should outweigh the risks. Then you verify the benefits and risks assessed individually before deciding on treatment for your patients based on the study results.

4.12 CASE REPORT # 12

4.12.1 How to Determine Whether or Not the Study That Proposes a New Diagnostic Test is Valid

With the development of new technology we have new diagnostic tests that become available for dosing the same biomarkers. Therefore, the health-care providers and others should be able to determine whether or not the study that proposes a new diagnostic test is valid. Also, the health-care provider should be able to determine if he/she can believe the results of the study and if the reported diagnostic accuracy is true.

Question # 1: Among the following, which are the elements that may help you decide whether or not the results are valid?

(A) Independent blind comparison with a reference standard;
(B) Patients sample representative of the population tested;
(C) Comparison with the reference standard;
(D) The methods for performing the test should be described in sufficient detail;
(E) All of the above are true.

Answer: **E**.

(A) Independent blind comparison with a reference standard: It is very important that those interpreting the results of the new diagnostic test should not be aware of the results of the reference test. Knowing the results of one study can influence how well the subsequent studies will be performed. Seeing the results of a CT scan may influence your ability to pick up an enlarged liver on a subsequent physical exam. To determine the accuracy of a test it must be compared with the "gold standard" for determining the diagnosis (liver biopsies). For instance, if you compared a new blood test for the diagnosis of prostate cancer with the PSA level then you would not know the accuracy of this test for this diagnosis of prostate cancer as PSA is not the more accurate test for the diagnosis of prostate cancer. However, if you compare the value of your new test with a prostate biopsy, which is the gold standard for the diagnosis of prostate cancer, then your new test will be more valid.

(B) Patients sample representative of the population tested: A given test is only valuable if it can distinguish between having and not having a disorder in the same population for which the test would be clinically useful. A blood test shown to be positive in 80% of a population of patients with ST-elevation myocardial infarct may not be useful in a general population of patients with chest pain. A more useful study might be to look at the blood test (for cardiac enzymes) in patients suspected of having a myocardial infarct.

(C) Comparison with the reference standard: The characteristics of the study test will change if the results influence whether or not a confirmatory test is performed. This "verification bias" can be problematic when the reference standard is invasive or harmful and clinicians are reluctant to have patients undergo a potentially harmful test. If only patients with a positive screening test for pulmonary embolism (PE) underwent pulmonary angiography then you would not know how many PEs were missed in the group that did not have angiography.

(D) The methods for performing the test should be described in sufficient details: To accept this criteria you must be able to replicate the exact test performed in the presented study to apply it to your patients. The technique for analysis and interpretation must be clearly described especially with more subjective tests.

Question # 2: What are the main elements that may help you decide about the relevance of the results?

(A) Likelihood ratio (LR);
(B) Sensitivity and specificity;
(C) A and B are important.

Answer: C.

(A) LR: The LR expresses the accuracy with which a diagnostic test identifies a disorder. The LR should be calculated for each level of a result if the test does not give a yes/no or positive/negative answer (such as with VQ scans [gold standard] in the case of pulmonary embolism). The LR tells you how likely a given test result correspond in patients with a disease compared with how likely the test result corresponds in patients without the disease. When calculating the LR (whether positive or negative) the proportion of patients with the disease will always be in the numerator and the proportion without the disease will be in the denominator. For instance, LR of 5 tells you that a given test results is 5 times more likely to occur in a patient with the disease as opposed to patients without the disease. In the contingency table below is an example of LR assessment on VQ scan and PE.

VQ Scan	PE Present	PE absent
Positive	150	250
Negative	35	750
Total	185	1000

LR+ = positive test in those with the disease/positive test in those without the disease
LR+ = (150/185)/(250/1000) = sensitivity/(1 − specificity) = 3.2
LR− = negative test in those with the disease/negative test in those without the disease
LR− = (35/185)/(750/1000) = (1 − sensitivity)/specificity = 0.25

How useful an LR is depends on how much it will raise or lower the pretest probability of the disorder. LRs > 1 increase the likelihood of a disorder and LRs < 1 decrease the likelihood of a disorder. In general, LRs less than or equal to 1 and LRs greater than 10 will be robust enough to significantly change the pretest probability. The easiest way to convert pretest probability to posttest probability is to use the Fagan nomogram (click here to use an interactive nomogram). Otherwise you need to convert the pretest probability to odds (probability/[1 − probability]) and multiply by the LR to get the posttest odds. The posttest odds can then be converted in probability (odds/[odds + 1]). By using LRs obviates the need for using sensitivity and specificity.

(B) Sensitivity and Specificity: Although the literature is moving toward reporting LRs, older studies will still put results in terms of sensitivity and specificity. Sensitivity is the proportion of patients with a disorder who have a positive test, and specificity is the proportion of patients without a disorder who have a negative test. A test with high sensitivity is useful for ruling out (Snout = "sensitivity rules out") a disorder, and a test with a high specificity is useful for ruling in (Spin = "specificity rules in") a disorder. These terms are more limiting than LRs because test results must be dichotomous or able to fit in a 2 × 2 table to calculate the sensitivity and the specificity.

Example of sensitivity and specificity from the above contingency table:

Sensitivity = proportion of patients with the disease who have a positive test
Sensitivity = 150/(150 + 35) = 150/185 = 81%
Specificity = proportion of patients without the disease who have a negative test
Specificity = 750/(250 + 750) = 750/1000 = 75%

Question # 3: True or False. After analyzing all the elements above, we should be able to answer whether or not the results help in taking care of your patients.

Answer: True.

A test must be reproducible in a defined clinical setting to be useful. If the test requires highly skilled individuals to interpret or observer disagreement is high, the test may be less useful outside of the study setting. Test properties can change in different subpopulations with more or less severe disease or in the presence of other conditions that influence the test result. You must compare your population of patients with the study population and examine the inclusion and exclusion criteria. If your patients are similar enough to the study population then you need to consider if the test result is robust enough to move your pretest probability to a posttest probability that would alter treatment. In other words, would the test result influence the management of an individual patient?

4.13 CASE REPORT # 13

4.13.1 How to Evaluate a Systematic Review or Meta-Analysis

Health-care professionals, professors, students, and others often use systematic review or metaanalysis to help them decide about a possible treatments or interventions. To achieve that, they need to ask themselves few important questions. We will use a recent study by Nour and Plourde to further clarify the concepts discussed in this case report (Unpublished data).

Question # 1: Among the following, which are the key questions that may help them decide whether or not these results would be useful for their patients?

(A) Did the authors of the systematic review or metaanalysis ask for a focused question?
(B) Are the inclusion criteria used to select the primary studies appropriate?
(C) Are there important relevant studies missing?
(D) Is the validity of primary studies examined?
(E) Is there a reproducible assessment of the primary studies?
(F) Are the results of the primary studies similar?
(G) All of the above are important.

Answer: G.

(A) Did the authors of the systematic review or metaanalysis ask for a focused question? The questions addressed by review articles usually pertain to certain patient populations undergoing treatment, a diagnostic test, or harmful exposure, and the associated outcome. The relevant question should be obvious from the title or the abstract of the article and be as specific as possible. For instance, Dr. Nour and Plourde performed a study measuring the role of physical activity for weight loss in obese adults. The item A is acceptable.

(B) Are the inclusion criteria used to select the primary studies appropriate? The specific criteria used to find primary studies should be outlined in the review article. This should include not only the patient population, exposure, and outcome of interest but also the methods for finding the primary studies such as a medline search using the terms of interest. With a vast database of studies such as medline, it is easy to find studies that will support preconceived conclusions. A good review will explicitly state inclusion criteria and include all appropriate articles regardless of outcome. For example in our study we searched from Medline, Scopus, and others and the following terms: exercise, physical activity, obesity, obesity-associated metabolic disorders, hypertension, type 2 diabetes mellitus, and others that are associated with obesity The systematic review was performed using the most recent article from the literature. The search respects the item B.

(C) Are there important relevant studies missing? The authors of reviews not only need to search databases such as medline but also examine article references and contact experts in the field to find unpublished or not yet referenced studies. Not everyone agrees on whether or not to include unpublished articles in reviews but not doing so increases the risk of "publication bias" in which only articles with positive outcomes are published. Because the authors are specialists in obesity, they got also the grey literature, unpublished data from their colleagues who are also specialist in obesity as well a summary (Abstract) of meeting on obesity. This was to ensure that no important articles were missing with positive or negative conclusions. Therefore, the item C is respected.

(D) Is the validity of primary studies examined? The strategy used to determine the validity of the primary studies should be stated and should be similar to the criteria that you would use in appraising original research. In a review of a new therapy, the methods for establishing validity of the primary studies should be the same as those used when looking at the studies individually. For our study, the validity of primary studies was determined using a specific algorithm (decision tree).

(E) Is there a reproducible assessment of the primary studies? Deciding the validity of studies is a subjective decision open to variability among investigators. Having more than one person analyze the primary studies to determine what to include in the review reduces errors and bias. This part of the study was performed with both coauthors (Nour and Plourde) who are also specialists in obesity, and after discussion both concurs on the selected articles.

(F) Are the results of primary studies similar? Most studies included in reviews have differences in patients, exposures, outcome measures, and research methods that make it difficult to compare the studies. There are statistical tests (tests of homogeneity) used in metaanalyses to determine whether the differences in results from study to study are due to chance alone. When there is statistically significant heterogeneity, it is less likely that differences in studies are due to chance and more likely that the studies are not measuring the same underlying effect and have important differences in patients, exposures, outcome measures, or research methods. A nonsignificant test does not rule out important differences between individual studies. The selection of our studies was performed using a heterogeneity test and only the most homogene studies were kept.

Question # 2: True of False. We should always question about the validity of the results.

Answer: True.

Reporting the number of positive and negative studies is not a reliable method for summarizing the results. Instead, primary studies are typically given more or less weight based on their size and quality. Reviews of treatment or prognostic factors often use OR to summarize the results. OR can be expressed as the odds of having an outcome in the exposed group divided by the odds of having an outcome in the control group or the odds that a patient with an adverse outcome was exposed divided by the odds that a control patient was exposed. If the outcome measures of different studies are not the same, the results of each study can be shown as "effect size" and then the effect sizes from each study can be combined. The effect size tells you how much difference there is between the control and intervention groups and is calculated by the difference in outcomes between the two groups divided by the standard deviation (SD). Although effect sizes are open to interpretation, an effect size of 0.8 is said to be a large effect (the two groups are separated by 0.8 SDs), 0.5 a moderate effect, and 0.2 a small effect. The size effect was highly acceptable (0.65 SDs) in the study by Nour and Plourde.

Question # 3: True or False. As for the other types of study, we should always be able to answer whether or not the results help in taking care of our patients.

Answer: True.

As for the previous questions you need to determine if the results are applicable to your patients. Look at the patient characteristics, subgroups, and inclusion and exclusion criteria to see if these match your patients. In a large review, there will more likely be a broad range of patients but the treatment may be more general than you would like. The results of our study demonstrated that physical activity is a good tool to make obese patients lose weight, but it is more efficient in combination with an adequate diet (strong recommendation; high-quality evidence using the grade system). Regular physical activity was helpful in improving the obesity-associated morbidity such as high blood pressure, type 2 diabetes, dyslipidemia, and others (strong recommendation; moderate-quality evidence). The results of this study have demonstrated that this treatment is useful for patients obese due to overconsumption of food, lack of physical activity, and bad dietary habits, i.e., for most patients seen in general practice setting (strong recommendations; moderate-quality evidence) But for obese patients having metabolic disorders the results of this study does not apply and these last patients should be seen by health specialists such as endocrinologists but not by general practitioners (weak recommendations; weak-quality evidence).

4.14 CASE REPORT # 14

4.14.1 How to Conduct a Case-Control Study

Abiraterone Acetate (Zytiga) is an antiandrogen drug recently put on the market for the treatment of metastatic prostate cancer. Based on the pre- and postmarketing studies, 30 cases of fatal liver failure have been published suggesting that Zytiga is associated with liver failure. Regarding this issue some researchers at Health Canada decided to conduct a case-control study to evaluate the association between Zytiga taken at 500 mg or 1000 mg per day and the risk of liver failure. The article will be entitled: Zytiga and the risk of liver failure and will be submitted to the BMJ.

Question # 1: Among the following, which are the key questions that may help the health-care providers assess the study design?

(A) Study hypothesis and sense;

(B) Selected study design;

(C) Comparison groups;

(D) How similar are these groups;

(E) Was the exposure clearly defined and capable of being reliably evaluated?

(F) Was the outcome clearly defined and capable of being reliably evaluated? Was it a clinically important outcome?

(G) Were the exposures and outcomes measured in the same way in the groups being compared?

(H) How good was follow-up? Was it appropriately long? Was there excessive loss to follow-up?

(I) All of the above are true.

Answer: I.

(A) Study hypothesis and sense: A hypothesis is never formally stated, although given the background of Zytiga and the case of liver failure, it could be assumed that the null hypothesis would be:

1. Among men, there is no association between liver failure and the use of Zytiga;
2. Among men, there is no association between the use of Zytiga (as either at 500 or 1000 mg/day) and liver failure.
3. Among men, there is no association between the duration of exposure to Zytiga and liver failure.

Studying the relationship between Zytiga and liver failure does make sense, given the published 30 case reports of an association between Zytiga and liver failure reported to Health Canada for the past 5 years. No prior studies on this topic with controls had been performed.

(B) Selected study design: As mentioned above, the investigators chose a case-control study design. The outcome of interest (liver failure) is rare, which makes this study design necessary. An RCT or cohort study would not have been logistically or ethically feasible. Furthermore, when the events of interest studied are rare, too much time and too many resources would be required to demonstrate significant trends in prospective cohort study.

(C) Comparison groups: Yes, there were cases ($n = 90$) and controls ($n = 177$). The authors were closed to achieving their goal of two controls/case (98% cases had two matched controls). They also achieved the number of patients needed to have a power of 80% to detect a statistically significant difference between cases and controls.

(D) How similar are these groups: The investigators did a perfect job collecting and reporting data on different patient characteristics. There were significant imbalances between the treated and the control groups where the treatment group was more often Caucasians and more educated. They were more likely to have a history of cancer and liver disease, recent use of Casodex (an antiandrogen drug) and a lower body mass index. As explained in the ICH E10, it is particularly relevant to have similar groups, this eliminate many difficulties when it will be time to interpret the results.

(E) Was the exposure clearly defined and capable of being reliably evaluated? The authors do not define the amount of Zytiga necessary to be considered an exposure. In terms of the time frame from exposure to outcome, the authors define a "window of exposure."(See Glossary of terms). The "window of exposure" essentially means exposure to Zytiga and the apparition of the onset of signs and symptoms that led to the diagnosis of liver failure. This "window of exposure" is defined as 4 months. The lack of an exposure is clearly defined as no use of Zytiga within the prior month. Exposure was determined as reliably as possible through live or phone interviews or by looking at the medical chart by trained researchers. Subjects were excluded if they could not communicate well enough by an interview within 30 days of the liver failure.

(F) Was the outcome clearly defined and capable of being reliably evaluated? Was it a clinically important outcome? The outcome was clearly defined as seen with liver enzyme or liver failure determined by liver biopsy. These findings are reliably evaluated, especially as the authors excluded any subjects with previous signs and symptoms of liver disease. Liver failure is a clinically important outcome due to its associated significant morbidity and mortality.

(G) Were the exposures and outcomes measured in the same way in the groups being compared? Exposures were measured in the same manner in both cases and controls. The outcome of interest, liver failure, occurred in only cases, so it was not measured in controls. Case-control studies in general are susceptible to recall bias and investigator bias (see Glossary of terms). The authors attempted to prevent recall bias by using a highly structured interview in which the subjects were blinded to the Zytiga hypothesis and interviewed within 30 days of the liver failure. (Although it is not clear that interviewing a shorter time after the outcome would decrease the tendency for recall bias.) Several strategies were used to reduce the possibility of selection bias: active case surveillance and objective determination of eligibility. Nine patients declined to participate (in two cases their primary-care providers refused their participation), so for the most part the patients selected were enrolled.

(H) How good was follow-up? Was it appropriately long? Was there excessive loss to follow-up? These questions only apply to RCTs and cohort studies as explained above.

Question # 2: Among the following, which are the key questions that may help the health-care providers assess the results?

(A) How strong was the association between exposure and outcome?
(B) Was there a temporal relationship between the exposure and outcome?
(C) Was there a dose-response gradient?
(D) How precise was the estimate of risk?

(E) Did the authors adjust for differences between comparison groups?
(F) Was the statistical analysis appropriate?
(G) All of the above are correct.

Answer: G.

(A) How strong was the association between exposure and outcome? The strength of inference will be less for this study because it had a case-control design and therefore there may have been confounding variables that were not recognized. The strength of association appears high and significant in men who had used Zytiga at 1000 mg/day (OR 7.2 (1.12−13.40) with $P = .04$). However, there was no association between the use of Zytiga at 500 mg/day and liver failure.

(B) Was there a temporal relationship between the exposure and outcome? The authors tried to establish this as much as they could by including as case patients only those who had taken Zytiga within 1 month of the liver failure. However, they do not mention what the duration of Zytiga use was in patients. Some patients taking Zytiga daily for years had a liver failure, which is quite different from someone who took it only for 1 month prior to their liver failure. The association between Zytiga exposure and liver failure would seem much greater in the second situation. They did perform a separate analysis of only patients who had been exposed to Zytiga after 1 month of their liver failure and found that adjusted ORs were slightly higher but still not statistically significant. The authors also mention the potential for temporal-precedence bias, which refers to a systematic error in which an exposure is counted although the exposure occurs after the onset of the disease under study, often in response to disease symptoms. One measure that the authors took to check for temporal-precedence bias was excluding all patients who had experienced an elevation of liver enzymes before taking Zytiga from the analysis. There was no major distortion of the results in doing so.

(C) Was there a dose-response gradient? The results of this study support a dose-response gradient. The investigators found the largest association of liver failure was at the highest dose of Zytiga. The authors also performed an analysis, which showed that the OR relating to liver failure and Zytiga was higher in those taking Zytiga 1000 mg per day, compared with those taking Zytiga 500 mg/day.

(D) How precise was the estimate of risk? The main "positive" result of the study was an OR of 7.2 for men using Zytiga 1000 mg/day acquiring liver failure. The 95% CI for this OR was 1.12−13.40, which is small (i.e., precise). However, the lower end of the CI, 1.12, is still above 1, so we can be convinced that there was a positive relationship. Men using 500 mg of Zytiga per day actually appeared to have a lower risk of liver failure (OR 0.62), which does not really make sense. The upper end of the CI (1.92) would suggest that we cannot exclude that men exposed to Zytiga 500 mg per day were at higher risk for liver failure. The bottom line is that a larger number of subjects might have produced more precise estimates of risk or no risk.

(E) Did the authors adjust for differences between comparison groups? Yes and no. It was observed that only the level of education changed the adjusted OR for the association with liver failure by more than 10%. The results were reported as adjusted for race, presence or absence of liver disease, and level of education. The authors did not adjust for a family history of liver disease, a lower body mass index, and/or recent exposure to Casodex because these entities did not change the adjusted OR by more than 10%. Together or separately, however, these could be confounding variables.

(F) Was the statistical analysis appropriate? Yes. First, the appropriate sample size required to show an association between Zytiga exposure and liver failure with 80% power was calculated. Chi-square and Fisher's exact tests were used to compare patient characteristics between groups. Conditional logistic models for matched sets were used to estimate ORs with CIs. They then calculated unadjusted and adjusted ORs.

Question # 3: True or False: Do you agree with the authors' conclusions?

Answer: True.

The conclusion that "among men between the ages of 50 and 75 years, the use of Zytiga at 1000 mg/day was associated with an increased risk of liver failure" is believable based on the study results. The authors mention numerous times that the use of Zytiga at 500 mg/day is likely to be associated with liver failure, although their data neither support nor negate these conclusions.

Question # 4: As for the questions above, should the results help in taking care of our patients or how applicable are the results? Among the following items, which one(s) help you answer that question?

(A) Did the risk apply to a narrow or broad population?
(B) What was the magnitude of the risk?
(C) Should clinical practice be altered because of the results of this study?
(D) All of the above are correct.

Answer: D.

(A) Did the risk apply to a narrow or broad population? The risk applied to men between the ages of 50–75 taking Zytiga. Which means that the risk of liver failure did not apply to a broader group of people.

(B) What was the magnitude of the risk? The magnitude of risk was estimated by the authors (Nour and Plourde) to be that 1 man may have a liver failure due to Zytiga within a 4 months window for every 50,000–1,268,000 men who use Zytiga at 1000 mg/day worldwide. The daily incidence of liver failure is of 0.6 per million for persons 50–75 years of age. Still this is only an estimate based on their OR and CI. This would seem clinically important given the estimate that millions of people taking Zytiga 1000 mg each month worldwide. Based on these estimates, at least 1–15 men would have a Zytiga-related liver failure a month or up to 100 Zytiga-related liver failure a year.

(C) Should clinical practice be altered because of the results of this study? There was a high strength of association (OR > 7) with a study design susceptible to unknown confounders and biases. Eliminating ~100 potential Zytiga-related liver failures a year would seem to be a mandate. Recommending patients not take Zytiga is not acceptable because this medication is the second-line hormone therapy for the treatment of hormone-resistant prostate cancer (advanced prostate cancer). Therefore, it seems unreasonable that the Health Canada and other regulatory agencies would recommend removing Zytiga from the market. Zytiga is now becoming more and more used. The main alternative health product Xtandi is not itself without potential health risks and is considered less efficient than Zytiga.

REFERENCES

1. Yates N, Lee DK, Maher M. Health Canada's progressive licensing framework. *CMAJ.* 2007;176:1845–1847.
2. Maher M. Legislative and regulatory modernization for therapeutic products. *J Popul Ther Clin Pharmacol.* 2010;17:E341–E348.
3. Heemstra HE, Giezen TJ, Mantel-Teeuwisse AK, de Vrueh RL, Leufkens H. Safety-related regulatory actions for orphan drugs in the US and EU: a cohort study. *Drug Saf.* 2010;33(2):127–137.
4. Gagne J, Thompson L, O'Keefe K, Kesselheim A. Innovative research methods for studying treatments for rare disease: methodological review. *BMJ.* 2014;349:g6802.
5. Plourde G. *Les Jeunes et l'obésité: Diagnostics et Interventions.* Presses de l'Université Laval; 2014.
6. Klein AV, Wang J, Bedford P. Subsequent entry biologics [biosimilars] in Canada: approaches to interchangeability and the extrapolation of indications and use. *GaBI J.* 2014;3:1–6.
7. Szarfman A, Machado SG, O'Neill RT. Use of screening algorithms and computer systems to efficiently signal higher-than-expected combinations of drugs and events in the US FDA's spontaneous report database. *Drug Saf.* 2002;25:381–392.
8. Almenoff JS, DuMouchel W, Kindman A, Yang X, Fram D. Disproportionality analysis using empirical Bayes data mining: a tool for the evaluation of drug interactions in the post-marketing setting. *Pharmacoepiedmiol Drug Saf.* 2003;12:517–521.
9. Glenny AM, Altman DG, Song F, et al. Indirect comparisons of competing interventions. *Health Technol Assess.* 2005;9:1–148.
10. Caldwell DM, Ades AE, Higgins JPT. Simultaneous comparison of multiple treatments: combining direct and indirect evidence. *BMJ.* 2005;331:897–900.
11. Bucher HC, Guyatt GH, Griffith LE, Walter SD. The results of direct and indirect treatment comparisons in meta-analysis of randomized controlled trials. *J Clin Epidemiol.* 1997;50:683–691.
12. Jansen JP, Crawford B, Bergman G, Stam W. Bayesian meta-analysis of multiple treatment comparisons: an introduction to mixed treatment comparisons. *Value Health.* 2008;11:956–964.

13. Cipriani A, Higgins JPT, Geddes JR, Salanti G. Conceptual and technical challenges in network meta-analysis. *Annals Intern Med.* 2013;159:130–137.
14. Kass RE. Statistical inference: the big picture. *Stat Sci.* 2011;26:1–9.
15. Song F, Xiong T, Parekh-Bhurke TS, et al. Inconsistency between direct and indirect comparisons of competing interventions: meta-epidemiological study. *BMJ.* 2011;343. Article ID d4909.

Chapter 5

Conclusion

As the title of this book suggests pharmacoepidemiology and pharmacovigilance work in synergy to allow for a better assessment and/or management of adverse drug reactions. Not too long ago, the clinical evaluation of drugs was mainly based on the results from randomized, controlled clinical trials; however, as we have shown in this book, the conclusions from clinical trials are limited to the patients enrolled in the trials. While the internal validity of these studies can be high, the external validity is not always representative of the drug's experience once used in the real world (i.e., uncontrolled settings). It has become increasingly necessary to complement data from experimental clinical trials data obtained in the real world of use of drugs in clinical practice (outside the context of clinical trials), i.e., throughout the entire life cycle of a product.

Pharmacovigilance is essentially based on the qualitative and quantitative study of spontaneous adverse drug reactions reports, followed by a clinical assessment/judgment with regards to its impact on the overall safety profile of the drug. It is particularly useful for identifying potential safety signals of a rare adverse event or in orphan disease settings where exposure data are limited prior to marketing. The purpose of pharmacovigilance is to enhance patient care and patient safety in relation to the use of medicines according to the life cycle of a health product. Furthermore, pharmacovigilance can support public health programs by providing ongoing data throughout a product's life cycle allowing for an accurate, reliable, and balanced assessment of the risk—benefit ratio of the product as more and more data becomes available with its use in the market.

Pharmacoepidemiology is best described as the study of drug use in real-world conditions in large populations to assess the effectiveness and risks associated with the use of a health product. Pharmacoepidemiology allows for the characterization of the conditions of use, misuse, clinical effectiveness, adverse drug reactions, and risks of drugs. The development of pharmacoepidemiology has allowed for a better optimization of drug uses. By studying larger populations in real-world settings, along with establishing reasonable comparable groups, pharmacoepidemiology studies allow for the quantification of risks that is impossible to carry out using spontaneous reporting alone. It also enables the highlighting and quantification of safety signals for events that are frequent and multifactorial, where the role of a drug in individual cases can be difficult to detect.

Pharmacoepidemiology and Pharmacovigilance. https://doi.org/10.1016/B978-0-12-816183-8.00005-6

Considering what it is mentioned in this book, we can confirm that the scientific disciplines of pharmacovigilance and pharmacoepidemiology truly complement one another and can be applied together to enhance drug safety, but in no way can one replace the other.

Annex 1

Glossary of Pharmacovigilance Terms

Adverse event (AE): This represents any unwanted medical incident in a patient or clinical trial participants administered a health product and which does not necessarily have to have a causal relationship with the treatment provided. An adverse event can therefore be any unfavorable sign including an abnormal laboratory finding, symptom, or health problem temporally associated with the use of a health product, whether or not considered related to the health product. An adverse event represents the frontline of the passive and active pharmacovigilance activities. For more information consult the guideline on Good Pharmacovigilance Practice by Health Canada.

Adverse event of special interest (AESI): This represents a specific event from a particular health product or class of products that a sponsor may wish to monitor carefully. It could be serious or nonserious (e.g., weight loss, incontinency, headaches, nausea, vomiting, and others) and could include events that might be the potential precursors or prodromes for more serious medical conditions in susceptible individuals. Such events should be described in the protocol or the protocol amendment, the investigator brochure (IB), and the product monograph when the health product is marketed, and instructions should be provided to the investigators on how and when they should report these adverse events to the sponsor. For more information consult the guideline on Good Pharmacovigilance Practice by Health Canada.

Adverse drug reaction (ADR): In the preapproval clinical experience with a new health product or for its new usages, particularly as the therapeutic dose(s) that may not be established, all noxious and unintended responses to a health product related to any dose should be considered adverse drug reactions. The phrase "due to a health product" means that a causal relationship between a health product and an adverse event is at least a reasonably or possibility related, i.e., the relationship cannot be ruled out (see Chapter 3 for a definition of these terms). Regarding the marketed health products, a well-accepted definition of an adverse drug reaction in the postmarketing setting reads as follows: A response to a health product which is noxious and unintended and which occurs at doses normally used in man for prophylaxis, diagnosis, or therapy of disease or for the modification of physiological function. For more information consult the guideline on Good Pharmacovigilance Practice by Health Canada.

Alert, warning: This represents a signal indicating a possible danger and implying need for appropriate action. In pharmacovigilance, this term is stronger than "signal" in that it indicates the existence of a risk that is quantitative and qualitative, whose significance is yet to be determined. An alert therefore justifies the implementation of a particular study (pharmacoepidemiology study) or suitable decision-making. For more information consult the guideline on Good Pharmacovigilance Practice by Health Canada.

Benefit–risk analysis: This is the essence of the approbation process by the regulatory agencies and consists in the examination of the favorable (beneficial) and unfavorable results of undertaking a specific course of action. While this expression is still commonly used, the more logical pairings of benefit/risk ratio is now replacing it.

Case noncase study: This is the method of analyzing a spontaneous reporting pharmacovigilance database using internal comparisons to investigate a possible association between the exposure to a health product and the occurrence of an adverse event (quantified by the calculation of a *relative reporting ratio*). However, this method cannot be a substitute for the classical epidemiological studies (i.e., cohort, case-control) but gives relatively reliable results if the database contains an almost infinite number of different drug–event combinations. This information is discussed in Chapter 3.

Case reports: This represents the report of an incidence in a single patient. As used in pharmacovigilance, a case report describes a single patient who was exposed to a health product and experiences a particular outcome, usually an adverse event.

Case series: Also being very important in pharmacovigilance activities, this term represents the reports of collections of patients, all of whom have a common exposure, examining what their clinical outcomes were. Alternatively, case series can be reports of patients who have a common disease, examining what their antecedent exposures were. In case series there is no control groups.

Clinical development program: This refers to all clinical trials being conducted with the same investigational drug, regardless of indication or formulation. The clinical development starts from the discovery of a new potential molecule and continues to the marketing of this health product. For the better example to explain the steps involved in the clinical development program please consult Fig. 1.1 of Chapter 1.

Clinical trial/study: This represents any investigation in human subjects put in place to discover or verify the clinical, pharmacological, and/or other pharmacodynamic effects of an investigational health product(s), and/or to identify any adverse reactions related to an investigational health product(s), and/or to study the absorption, distribution, metabolism, and excretion

(ADME) (pharmacokinetic) of an investigational health product(s) with the object of ascertaining its safety and/or efficacy, i.e., its benefit/risk ratio. This term will be further discussed in Chapter 3.

Cohort studies: This term represents the studies that identify defined populations and follow them forward in time, examining their rates of disease. The cohort studies generally identify and compare exposed patients to unexposed patients or to patients who receive a different exposure. The definition of cohort study will be further explained in Chapter 3 that discuss pharmacoepidemiology in the management of adverse drug reactions.

Company core safety information (CCSI): This document represents for health products; all relevant safety information contained in the company core data sheet prepared by the marketing authorization holder (MAH) or the sponsor and which the MAH requires to be listed in all countries where the company is marketing the product, except when the local regulatory authority specifically requires a modification.

Company core data sheet (CCDS): This document represents for health products, a document prepared by the MAH containing, in addition to safety information, material related to the indications, dosing, pharmacology, and other information concerning the health product that might guide the prescriber on the appropriate and safer use of the product. This document might be comparable for all countries where this product is marketed.

Cross-sectional studies: This kind of study examines exposures and outcomes in populations at one point in time. The purpose of this type of study will be further explained in Chapter 3 that discusses more in depth the studies related to pharmacoepidemiology; the other important partner involved in a better management of adverse drug reactions The cross-sectional studies are very useful for the pharmacovigilance activities as it helps establishing the background information for various diseases, risk factors, and others.

Data Monitoring Committee (synonyms: Independent Data Monitoring Committee, Data and Safety Monitoring Board): This is an independent data monitoring committee that may be established by the sponsor to assess at time intervals the progress of a clinical trial, the safety data, and the critical efficacy endpoints and to recommend to the sponsor whether to continue, modify, or stop a trial. For further information on the data monitoring committee please consult the ICH-E6 on Good Clinical Practice and the Food and Drug Laws and Regulations. See Annex 3 at the end of this book.

Descriptive studies: This term represents studies that do not have control groups, namely case reports, case series, and analyses of secular trends. They contrast with analytic studies. However, we used them to obtained baseline information for the populations under studies. Again, this term will be further discussed in Chapter 3.

Drug utilization research: This term represents the marketing, distribution, prescription, and use of drugs in a society, with special emphasis on the resulting medical, social, and economic consequences. Although, not documented in the text, this is very useful for the active surveillance of adverse drug reactions.

Expected adverse drug reaction: This term represents an adverse drug reaction for which its nature or severity is consistent with that included in the appropriate reference safety information (e.g., investigator's brochure for an unapproved investigational product or package insert, summary of product characteristics, or the Canadian product monograph for an approved health product).

Good clinical practice (GCP): This is a standard guideline for the design, conduct, performance, monitoring, auditing, recording, analyses, and reporting of clinical trials adverse drug reactions that provides assurance that the data and reported results are credible and accurate and that the rights, integrity, and confidentiality of trial subjects are protected. This is an important component of the product life cycle discussed in Fig. 1.1 of Chapter 1. It is an important concept promoted by the ICH-E6 on Good Clinical Practice and part of the Food and Drug Laws and Regulations.

Good pharmacovigilance practice: This is a set of guidelines for the conduct of pharmacovigilance in Canada and other countries including the United States, the EU, and others in cooperation with competent authorities in Member States and interested parties and applying to MAH worldwide. This is an important component of the product life cycle discussed in Fig. 1.1. It is an important concept promoted by the ICH-E8 on Good Pharmacovigilance Practice and part of the Food and Drug Laws and Regulations.

Harm (synonymous with adverse drug reaction): This term is an important term in drug safety and represents the totality of possible adverse consequences of an intervention or therapy; they are the direct opposite of benefits, against which they must be compared. The damage is qualified by measures of frequency of occurrence, severity, or duration. They represent the nature and extent of actual damage that could be caused by a health product. They should not to be confused with risk. The important concept of number needed to harm will be discussed at the next chapter to consolidate the information on harm.

Identified risk: This consists in an unwanted incident for which there is adequate evidence of an association with the health product of interest. Examples of identified risks include: an adverse reaction adequately demonstrated in nonclinical studies and confirmed by clinical data; an adverse reaction observed in well-designed clinical trials or epidemiological studies for which the magnitude of the difference is compared with the comparator group (placebo or active substance) on a parameter of interest suggesting a causal relationship; and an adverse drug reaction suggested by a number of well-documented spontaneous reports where causality is strongly supported by temporal relationship and biological plausibility, such as anaphylactic reactions, application site reactions, and others.

Important identified risk, important potential risk: This represents an identified risk or potential risk that could impact the benefit/risk ratio of health product or have implications for public health. What constitutes an important risk will depend on several factors, including the impact on the individual, the seriousness of the risk, and the impact on public health. Normally, any risk that is likely to be included in the contraindications or warnings and precautions section of the product labeling should be considered important identified and potential risk.

International Classification of Diseases (ICD): This is the classification of diseases proposed by the World Health Organization (WHO). It is used in most databases to code diseases or reasons for practitioner consultation.

International Conference on Harmonization (ICH): This term involves the process of implicating the European, US, and Japanese regulatory authorities and pharmaceutical industry associations to promote the development of harmonious regulation for drug registration. There are three main areas (quality, safety, and efficacy) with many subtopics, many of which have been incorporated into national or community regulations. Although mainly focused on premarketing activities, there are some topics that also concern pharmacovigilance. Health Canada complies with these harmonization rules.

Investigator brochure (IB): This document consists in a compilation of the clinical and nonclinical data on the health product(s) that is relevant to the study of the investigational product(s) in human subjects. This IB should be regularly updated to ensure that the investigators remained well informed about new important identified risk or important potential risks.

Investigational product: This term consists in a pharmaceutical or biological form of an active ingredient or placebo being tested or used as a reference in a clinical trial, including a health product with a marketing authorization when used or assembled (formulated or packaged) in a way different from the approved form, or when used for an unapproved indication (off-label), or when used to gain further information about an approved use.

Labeled or unlabeled: For a health product with an approved marketing application, any reaction that is not mentioned in the official product information is unlabeled. If it is included it is termed labeled. For example, any reactions included in the Canadian product monograph are considered labeled.

Mandatory reporting: This is a legal obligation for a health-care professional who has observed an adverse drug reaction to notify a pharmacovigilance system. It has not been demonstrated that making reporting mandatory changes reporting rates or patterns.

Medication errors: This is an important term to consider in pharmacoepidemiology and other studies and represents any mistake in the health product use process, including prescribing, transcribing, dispensing, administering, and monitoring. The investigator should remain aware of this possibility as it could impact the validity of a trial and the safety of clinical trial participants or the patient when the product is marketed.

Minimum criteria for reporting: For the purpose of reporting cases of suspected adverse drug reactions, the minimum data elements for a case are: an identifiable reporter, an identifiable patient and his/her medical history, an adverse reaction, and a suspect health product. A good reporting of adverse drug reactions is particularly important as if forms the basis for passive and active surveillance.

Missing information: This represents the gaps in knowledge about a health product, related to safety or use in particular patient populations, which could be clinically significant in the interpretation of data. For more information, please consult the ICH-E9 on statistical procedure for clinical research available at the Resources for the Readers section in Annex 4.

Pharmacovigilance system: This consists in a system used by regulatory authorities such as Health Canada, the FDA, the EMA, and others to fulfill its legal tasks and responsibilities in relation to pharmacovigilance and to the monitoring of safety about authorized health products and to detect any change to their benefit/risk ratio.

Postauthorization safety study (PASS): This term represents any study relating to an authorized health product conducted with the aim of identifying, characterizing or quantifying a safety hazard, of confirming the safety profile of the health product, or of measuring the effectiveness of risk management measures. This is a good example of active surveillance of adverse drug reactions.

Potential risk: This term consists in an unwanted incident for which there is some basis for suspicion of an association with the health product of interest but where this association has not been confirmed. Examples of potential risks include: nonclinical safety concerns that have not been observed or resolved in clinical studies; adverse events observed in clinical trials or epidemiological studies for which the magnitude of the difference, compared with the comparator group (placebo or active substance, or unexposed group), on the parameter of interest raises a suspicion of, but is not large enough to suggest, a causal relationship; an event that is known to be associated with other products of the same class or which could be expected to occur based on the properties of the health product. For more information consult the guideline on Good Pharmacovigilance Practice by Health Canada.

Prescription event monitoring (PEM): This represents a postmarketing surveillance tool, based on a follow-up of the first prescription of selected new drug. This is a useful method for active pharmacovigilance.

Reference safety information (RSI): In periodic benefit–risk ratio evaluation reports (see above in Chapter 2) for any health products, all relevant safety information contained in the reference product information (e.g., the company core data sheet) prepared by the MAH and which the MAH requires to be listed in all countries where it markets the health product, except when the local regulatory authority specifically requires a modification.

Risk–benefit balance: This term represents an evaluation of the positive therapeutic effects (efficacy) of the health product in relation to the risks (safety), i.e., any risk relating to the quality, safety, or efficacy of the health product in regards to the patients' health or public health.

Safety concern: This term represents an important identified risk, an important potential risk, or important missing information. It is noted that the ICH E2A definition of safety concern an important identified risk, an important potential risk, or important missing information, i.e., includes the qualifier "important" in relation to missing information.

Serious adverse event (SAE): This important term represents an unwanted medical incident that at any dose, results in death, is life threatening, requires inpatient hospitalization or prolongation of existing hospitalization, results in persistent or significant disability/incapacity, or is a congenital anomaly/birth defect. A medical and scientific judgment should be exercised in deciding whether other situations should be considered serious such as important medical events that might not be immediately life threatening or result in death or hospitalization but might jeopardize the patient or might require intervention to prevent one of the other outcomes listed in the definition above. Examples of such events are intensive treatment in an emergency room or at home for allergic bronchospasm, blood dyscrasias, or convulsions that do not result in hospitalization, or development of drug dependency or drug abuse. For more information consult the ICH-E2A guidelines.

Side effect: This term represents any unwanted effect of a pharmaceutical or biological product occurring at normal dosage, which is related to the pharmacological properties of the health product.

Signal: This term consists in the information that arises from one or multiple sources (including observational or experimental studies), that suggests a new potentially causal association, or a new aspect of a known association, between an intervention and an event or set of related events, either adverse or beneficial, that is judged to have a sufficient likelihood to justify further action to verify. A signal may also refer to new information on an already-known association. Usually more than a single report is required to generate a signal, depending on the seriousness of the event and the quality of the information. See Chapter 4 for good concrete examples of signal.

Signal management process: This process includes the following activities: signal detection, signal validation, signal confirmation, signal analysis and prioritization, signal assessment, and recommendation for action. It is therefore a set of activities performed to determine whether, based on an examination of individual case safety reports, aggregated data from active surveillance systems or studies, literature information or other data sources, that there are new risks causally associated with an active substance or a health product or whether known risks have changed. See Chapter 4 for good concrete examples of signal.

Signal validation: This process consists in the evaluating of the data supporting a detected signal to verify that the available documentation contains sufficient evidence demonstrating the existence of a new potentially causal association, or a new aspect of a known association, and therefore justifies further analysis of the signal.

Solicited reports: Those solicited reports derived from organized data collection systems, which include clinical trials, registries, other patient support and disease management programs, surveys of patients or health-care providers, or information gathering on efficacy or patient compliance. These solicited reports are often used in the active surveillance of adverse drug reactions. For more information consult the guideline on Good Pharmacovigilance Practice by Health Canada.

Spontaneous reporting: This is a mean of passive surveillance based on the collection, usually on a national level, of cases of an adverse effect associated with marketed drugs. The surveyed population theoretically includes all of the patients treated by the health product in the geographic region considered. In spontaneous reporting, the observer of an adverse effect is expected to report it to a clearly and adequately documented and, if possible, a unique surveillance system. This assumes that the observer identifies the adverse effect, is aware of the existence of the surveillance system, and is convinced of the need to report adverse effects that he or she observes. The method thus rests on the motivation of the observer (hence the term "*spontaneous*") and is therefore subject to numerous biases, notably, selection bias. The reporting of adverse effects is "volunteer" in many countries; this rarely ensures exhaustive collection of all the adverse events that have occurred with a specific health product. Moreover, it gives no direct information on the size or characteristics of the population treated with the drug, or the treatment conditions (dose, duration, associated drug use, etc.), which makes it difficult to calculate an incidence rate or to detect risk factors. Spontaneous reporting is, however, quite irreplaceable as a means to detect previously unknown adverse effects (i.e., as an alert system). In certain situations the surveillance method can be based on less random information gathering, for example, by sending reporting forms to prescribers, making regular calls or visits to these prescribers, or setting up a computerized network. The term *spontaneous reporting* should, however, be retained to denote any prospective population surveillance method, which does not ensure exhaustive collection of cases and which gives no information on the size or characteristics of the exposed population.

Stimulated reporting: This can occur in certain situations, such as after a direct health-care professional communication, communication to hospitals, patient communication or a publication in the press or after a questioning of health-care professionals by company representatives. The adverse reaction reports arising from these situations are considered spontaneous reports, provided the report meets the definition of a spontaneous report as specified above. Reporting can also be stimulated by invitation from patients' or consumers' organizations to their members. Reporting can also be made in the context of early phase postmarketing surveillance.

Target population (treatment): This represents the patients who might be treated with the health product in accordance with the indication(s) and contraindications in the authorized product information such as the investigator brochure or the Canadian product monograph.

Unexpected adverse drug reaction: This consists in an adverse reaction where the nature or severity of which is not consistent with the applicable product information (e.g., investigator's brochure for an unapproved investigational health product). An adverse drug reaction whose nature, severity, specificity, or outcome is not consistent with the term or description used in the local/regional product labeling (e.g., package insert, summary of product characteristics, or Canadian product monograph) should be considered unexpected.

Validated signal: This represents a signal that contains sufficient evidence to demonstrate the existence of a new potentially causal association, or a new aspect of a known association, and therefore justifies further analysis of the signal. Chapter 4 provides concrete examples of signal analysis.

REFERENCES

Begaud B. *Dictionary of Pharmacoepidemiology*. John Wiley & Sons Ltd; 2000.

CIOMS Working Group Pharmacovigilance (2016). Available at: https://cioms.ch/pharmacovigilance/becoming-the-cioms-member/.

Health Canada: Good Pharmacovigilance Practices (GVP) Guidelines (GUI-0102) (2013). Available at: https://www.canada.ca/content/dam/hc-sc/migration/hc-sc/dhp-mps/alt_formats/pdf/compli-conform/gmp-bpf/docs/gui-0102_gvp-eng.pdf.

ICH guideline E2B (R3) on electronic transmission of individual case safety reports (ICSRs) - data elements and message specification - implementation guide (2013). Available at: http://www.ema.europa.eu/docs/en_GB/document_library/Scientific_guideline/2009/09/WC500002767.pdf.

ICH Topic E 3: Structure and Content of Clinical Study Reports (1996). Available at: http://www.ema.europa.eu/docs/en_GB/document_library/Scientific_guideline/2009/09/WC500002832.pdf.

ICH Harmonized Tripartite Guideline. Guideline for Good Clinical Practice E6 (R1); 1996. Available at: http://www.ich.org/fileadmin/Public_Web_Site/ICH_Products/Guidelines/Efficacy/E6_R1/Step4/E6_R1__Guideline.pdf.

ICH Harmonized Tripartite Guideline. Choice of Control Group and Related Issues in Clinical Trials (E10); 2000. Available at: www.ich.org//choice-ofcontrol-group-and-related-issues-in-clinical-trials.pdf.

ICH Harmonized Tripartite Guideline. Clinical Safety Data Management: Definitions and Standards for Expedited Reporting E2A; 1994. Disponible à http://www.ich.org/fileadmin/Public_Web_Site/ICH_Products/Guidelines/Efficacy/E2A/Step4/E2A_Guideline.pdf.

Samet JM, Wipfli H, Platz EA, Bavspar N. A Dictionary of Epidemiology. In: Porta Miquel, ed. *American Journal of Epidemiology*. Fifth Edition 170. 2009:1449.

World Health Organization. Available at: http://www.who.int/topics/epidemiology/en/.

Annex 2

Glossary of Pharmacoepidemiology Terms

Absolute risk: This term represents the risk measured in a population exposed to the factor of interest. The absolute risk adds the risk for this population if they have not been exposed (*background risk*, *reference risk*) and the risk induced by exposure (*excess risk*, *attributable risk*). This term has also been defined in the text of Chapter 3 and explained by concrete examples in Chapter 4.

Active ingredient: This adjective is applied to a health product if its administration to a living organism induces or could induce one or more pharmacodynamic effect(s). The activity from this ingredient does not necessarily imply a therapeutic effect. There are substances that induce one or more pharmacodynamic effect(s), without any therapeutic action or active principle: Active ingredient can also be defined as a substance responsible for some or all of the real or expected effects of a health product.

Additive: This term is used when the association of two or more factors produces an effect equal to the sum of the effects of each of the factors used alone. This term is used in pharmacology for interactions between two or more health products. This term is also referring to the sum of their therapeutic or undesirable effects, and in epidemiology, it refers to the sum of the effects or risks induced by each of the factors.

Ad hoc study: This is a kind of study conceived specifically for a precise objective, generally to answer a single concern raised by the regulatory agency. The ad hoc studies are contrasted in this respect with multipurpose studies, which attempt to answer several, sometimes very different, concerns and with the reanalyses of data previously collected for other purposes. This kind of study could be asked by a Regulatory Agency in case where safety concerns are identified. See article C.01. 019 from the Food Drugs and Regulations in the annex 3 at the end of this book.

Adjustment: This is a procedure having the goal to minimize or eliminate the effect of differences in the distribution of one or more variables. An adjustment is particularly important when those variables may act as confounders when studying the causal association between exposure to a given factor and the occurrence of an adverse event. An adjustment always takes place during an analysis, that is, subsequent to data collection. In this way, an incidence rate, relative risk, or odds ratio are said to be *adjusted* for a given variable, e.g., age, sex, body mass index, if its calculation took into account the possible differences in the distribution of this variable in the compared populations (see text for more information). An adjustment may use several statistical methods, such as the logistic regression model, or the covariance analysis. If the interfering variable has a large influence, the value of the adjusted parameter may differ markedly from the unadjusted value.

Admission bias, referral bias: This kind of bias has already been discussed in the text (see Chapter 3). We found useful to consolidate the information surrounding this topic as they are particularly relevant. Therefore, we decided to briefly discuss this issue here. A selection bias is that in which a subject has a different probability of being hospitalized or admitted to a healthcare system participating in recruiting study subjects, according to whether the person does or does not present a characteristic linked to the parameter to be measured. The parameter may thus be over- or underrepresented in the study sample compared to the source population, which will bias the measurement. This type of bias can alter the estimates made from cohort or case-control studies.

Adverse drug reaction, adverse reaction, and adverse effect: This is an important term that represents a response to a health product that is noxious and unintended and occurs at doses normally used in human for the prophylaxis, diagnosis, or for the therapy of disease (treatment) or for the modification of physiological function. The definition excludes the events related to accidental or deliberate overdose. Unlike "adverse event," the term "adverse drug reaction" implies that a causal relationship with the treatment was ascertained or is strongly suspected (see text for a definition of causality assessment). Then these adverse drug reactions can be categorized as expected or unexpected. Please also consult the previous glossary of pharmacovigilance terms as it contains relevant information of this issue and others terms that could also be related to pharmacoepidemiology.

Alternative hypothesis: This is a priori specified hypothesis that is accepted when the null hypothesis is rejected by statistical testing.

Anatomical Therapeutical Chemical Classification (ATC): This term represents the international health product classification proposed by the WHO Collaborating Centre for Drug Statistics Methodology, originally elaborated by the Nordic Council on Medicine, Oslo, Norway. Its initial goal was to compare drug utilization between countries in conjunction with the defined daily doses. It has since become the reference health product classification, even for other purposes.

Assessment, evaluation: This is an important term that consists in estimating or appraising the value of a parameter, a health product, or a treatment strategy as a function of pertinent and generally predefined criteria, considering all of the available data. In this way, the new drug approval (NDA) commission of a regulatory agency evaluates the risk/benefit ratio of new health products on the basis of all of the preclinical and clinical trials and according to standardized criteria. The term *assessment* also represents the result of such an evaluation.

Association, correlation, statistical dependence: This represents the probable statistical relationship observed between two or more variables. *For example, there is an association if the probability of occurrence of an event (or the number of cases of an event) varies as a function of the presence or the absence of a variable or due to the value of that variable.* An association is said to be *positive* if the probability of an event's occurrence is greater in the presence of a specific factor, or if the values of two variables tend in the same direction. An association is defined to be *negative* if the probability of an event's occurrence is smaller in the presence of a factor, or if the values of two variables tend in opposite directions. Although one may speak of *fortuitous association* (i.e., explained only by chance), the term "association" is generally reserved for a statistically significant relationships. This significance, however, does not necessarily imply the existence of a causal relationship between the variable in question and the measured parameter.

Antagonism: It is the values of two variables that tend in opposite directions. Although one may speak of *fortuitous association* (i.e., explained only by chance), the term 'association' is generally reserved for statistically significant relationships. As mentioned above, this significance, however, does not necessarily imply the existence of a causal relationship between the variable in question and the measured parameter.

Attack rate: This represents the cumulative incidence rate usually measured over a short period of time and often used to describe an epidemic. More information about the attack rate is available in Chapter 3.

Attributable: This is an adjective that may be accounted for by exposure to a risk factor, or to a health product treatment. *Example: A majority of cases of headache occurring in these patients were attributable to their cancer treatment of the cancer itself.*

Attributable fraction of the risk in the exposed: This represents the proportion of exposed cases for which the occurrence of the event of interest is attributable to exposure. The fraction thus indicates the proportion by which the risk of the event measured in an exposed population would be reduced were the exposure is eliminated. The attributable fraction of the risk (*AFR*) is calculated by dividing the risk difference between the exposed and the nonexposed by the risk measured in the exposed. For more information please consult the text in Chapter 3.

Attributable fraction of the risk in the population: This term consist in the proportion of cases of an event observed in a defined population (region, country, town, etc.) attributable to the exposure of a part of this population to a given factor. The attributable fraction thus indicates the proportion by which the risk of the event would be reduced in this population were the exposure is eliminated. The attributable fraction of the risk (*AFR*) is calculated by dividing the difference between the risk of the event in the entire population and the risk measured in the nonexposed subjects of the population by the risk in the entire population. In a public health context, this parameter allows estimation of the proportion of cases of a given event or illness, which could be avoided by the elimination of a risk factor (e.g., the withdrawal of a health product from the market). *Example: If the relative risk of Progressive Multifocal Leukoencephalopathy (PML) associated with the use of a Rituxan is 5% and if 1% of the population is exposed to this drug, the attributable fraction of the risk in this population is 0.004. This means that 4.0% of the cases of PML occurring in this population are attributable to Rituxan and would therefore be avoided if exposure to this health product is eliminated.* This type of estimate is only valid if the characteristics of the exposed and nonexposed subjects in the population are identical to those of the subjects who were compared for the relative risk or odds ratio calculation (see text). The definition and the conditions of exposure (dose, duration, etc.) are identical to those that were present for the relative risk calculation.

Attributable number of cases: This represents the number of cases of an event whose occurrence in a population is related to exposure to a given risk factor.

Attrition: This term is describing the fact that in a prospective study a certain number of subjects leave the study before the planned end of the follow-up, for various reasons such as death, lost to follow-up, intercurrent diseases, and others. Attrition is most often expressed as a percentage. *For example, if 200 subjects out of the 5000 included in a cohort study were not followed until the end of the term anticipated in the protocol, the attrition percentage is (200/5000) × 100% = 4.0%.* In pharmacoepidemiology, it is important to control the phenomenon of attrition, which can not only lead to a loss of statistical power, in the quantitative sense, but can also introduce significant bias if the attrition is linked to the phenomenon being studied (exposed vs. nonexposed).

Background noise: This term may apply, for example, to the incidence of an event in the general population or in a reference population. When this noise is high, the substantial number of coincidental associations expected during a follow-up may make it difficult to detect a moderately increased risk associated with an exposure. In the case of surveillance by spontaneous reporting (passive surveillance), background noise is formed by all cases (varying greatly in type, seriousness, and validity) reported for a given health product.

Baseline risk, background risk: This is an important information for the initiation of many clinical studies and represents the risk measured in a population not exposed to the factor under study. This term is often used to designate a risk estimated in the general population when, in fact, it more accurately represents a reference risk (measured in a population identical to the exposed population in all aspects except for the exposure status). Knowing this information is very relevant when you performed pharmacoepidemiologic studies.

Bayes's theorem: This represents the first mathematical formulation, by the Reverend Thomas Bayes (1702–61), of the principle of conditional probabilities allowing calculation of the probability that an event will occur or that an affirmation will be correct under certain conditions (e.g., that a test is positive or negative, or that a symptom is present or absent). In this formulation, the odds of presenting the disease given a positive test (*posterior odds*) is equal to the odds of presenting the disease estimated before analysis (*prior odds*) multiplied by the odds that the test will be positive if the disease is present. The multiplier of the prior odds is called the *likelihood ratio.* Bayes' theorem has numerous applications in clinical and epidemiological research. Among other uses, it has been applied to causality assessment in individual cases (see Chapters 3 and 4). The principle consists of fixing, before analysis, the prior odds that the health product of interest is responsible for the adverse event observed in a given patient. These odds are 1 if there is no reason to favor the hypothesis of the responsibility or non-responsibility of the health product for the adverse event. In the most favorable cases, the prior odds can be estimated from the relative risk or odds ratio quantified by a previous epidemiological study. The prior odds are then multiplied by one or more likelihood ratio(s) corresponding to available information, signs, or available criteria relevant to the causality analysis. Each likelihood ratio is calculated by dividing the probability of the criterion being present, if the health product is responsible for the event, by the probability of the criterion being present if the health product is not responsible. *Example: If 65% of patients presenting a given adverse effect are female when the proportion of females among all users of a health product of interest is 45%, the likelihood ratio for the gender will be 0.65/0.45 = 1.4.* The multiplication of the prior odds by all the likelihood ratios relevant for the causality analysis gives the final or posterior odds that the health product is responsible for the adverse event of interest. As explained in the text this theorem is highly useful when we performed a disproportional analysis in the assessment of specific adverse events associated with a health product (see text in Chapters 3 and 4).

Benefit: This important word is associated with the determination of the benefit/risk ratio where the benefit usually refers to a gain (positive result) for an individual or a population resulting from an intervention, i.e., a health product treatment. The expected benefit can be expressed quantitatively, and this would ordinarily incorporate an estimate of the probability of achieving the gain. In pharmacology, the term benefit is often used to estimate the efficacy of a treatment and if we also calculate the risk, this expression will become the risk/benefit ratio. Very importantly, when a regulatory agency decides to authorize a health product for marketing, these benefits should outweigh the risk (favorable risk/benefit ratio).

Berkson's bias: This represents a particular form of admission bias that can falsify an estimate made in a case-control study. This bias can occur if the cases are identified in a care structure and there is a higher (or a lower) probability that a case will be referred to this structure if exposed to the factor of interest. The strength of the association between exposure and an event can thus be artificially increased (or decreased). *Example: If, in a case-control study evaluating the association between the use of a health product and heart injury, the cases were selected in a cardiology department specialized in heart injury caused by medications, the probability of exposure of the cases to a particular health product may be abnormally high, which may lead to the conclusion of a stronger association than that which exists in reality. The effect would be the opposite if cases of heart injury of unknown cause were preferentially hospitalized. Health product known to be cardiotoxic could be underrepresented in this sample of hospital cases.*

Beta error: See Type II error.

Bias: This important term in epidemiological research represents an error of reasoning or procedure leading to a false representation of reality. In the regulatory sense, bias is systematic in nature and alters estimation in a given direction. Bias is thus different from *random error*, which results in a loss of precision but not in systematic deviation in a given direction. A particular kind of bias, called *confounding*, can be taken into account or corrected for during the analysis. Other biases known as selection and information biases alter the relevance or the validity of the collected data and cannot be subsequently controlled for in the analysis. The principal biases mentioned in this glossary of pharmacoepidemiologic terms can be grouped into three categories: *Selection biases*: admission bias, Berkson's bias, diagnostic bias, notoriety bias, and survival bias; *Information biases*: interviewer bias and recall bias; and *Interpretation biases*: aggregation bias, confounding, prescription bias (confounding by indication), protopathic bias, and reverse causality bias. The impacts played by these biases in pharmacoepidemiology studies are further discussed in Chapter 3, in the section discussing bias.

Binary variable: This sort of variable may only take two values (e.g., 0 or 1, diseased or nondiseased, alive or dead, male or female, and others). To simplify the analysis, certain continuous quantitative variables (e.g., weight, height, blood glucose, serum creatinine, and others) may be transformed into binary variables by fixing a cut-off value. For example, the subjects of a study can be divided into two groups: those with a BMI of less than 30 kg/m^2 (1) and those with a value of 30 kg/m^2 or higher (2).

Binomial distribution, binomial law: It is a kind of law describing the distribution of the probability of observing x successes over n independent tests, assuming that for each test there is an identical probability p of success. The outcome of each test must be binary (success/failure, diseased/nondiseased, alive/dead, and others). The binomial law thus describes a probability distribution that is discrete or discontinuous. In pharmacoepidemiology, the binomial distribution is used to calculate the probability of observing a given number of events x in a sample of size n; the exposure of each of the n subjects to the health product is considered as an independent test. The binomial distribution assumes that the probability p of the occurrence of the event is identical for each of the n subjects.

Biosimilar biologic drug or biosimilar: This is a kind of drug demonstrated to be highly similar to a biologic drug that was already authorized for sale (known as the *reference biologic drug*). Biosimilars were previously known in Canada as subsequent entry biologics (SEBs). Biosimilars are approved based on a thorough comparison to a reference health product and may enter the market after the expiry of reference drug patents and data protection.

Blinding: This is an important biostatistics terms used in clinical research and is used to demonstrate the ignorance of the fact or nature of exposure of a subject or group, which is planned and organized in the protocol of a study, to avoid the direct or indirect influence of such knowledge on the planned evaluation. A standard use of blinding is in controlled clinical trials. In a single-blind clinical trial, either the patient or the researcher does not know the type of treatment used (i.e., the health product of interest or an active or inactive referent); in a double-blind clinical trial, neither the researcher nor the patient know the nature of the treatment received by the latter; in a triple-blind clinical trial, in addition, the statistical analysis is conducted before the blinding codes are opened, thus without knowledge of the nature of the compared treatments. Implementation of blinding generally requires the preparation of pharmaceutical forms specific to the trial, perfectly identical in their presentation, whose only difference (which should be undetectable during the study) is the nature of the ingredients (e.g., active or inactive, placebo or real ingredients). The treatments are identified by a code known only by the organizer of the trial, which is opened at the end of the study period, or before if required by safety concerns. Blinding is also used in pharmacoepidemiology, for example during the validation leading to the inclusion of a case in a case-control study, to avoid the situation in which knowledge of the subject's exposure status influences the judgment of the investigators.

Carryover effect: This kind of error consists of not attributing an event or effect to an earlier exposure whose influence on the organism persists despite cessation of the exposure. The carry-over may be due to the persistence of significant concentrations of the health product in the organism or to lasting biological modifications induced by the treatment. Carryover effect is of particular concern in studies that compare the effect of several successive treatments, as well as in studies or trials in which the subject is his or her own control (crossover studies or trials). This phenomenon can be avoided by separating treatment periods being compared by sufficiently long intervals without treatment (*washout periods*) (see below).

Case: This qualifies any person or event presenting the characteristic(s) defined as the object(s) of interest for a study.

Case-cohort study: This represents an epidemiological design in which the population of subjects having presented an event during the follow-up of a cohort is compared, with respect to an exposure at baseline, with a control population chosen at random from the whole population of subjects present at the beginning of this period (see text under this subtitle in Chapter 3 for further information). Because of this mode of selection, the control population may include one or more subject(s) who will eventually become cases. Case-cohort studies differ from nested case-control studies in that controls, in the former, are not matched to the cases within the cohort but selected randomly at the beginning of the follow-up. This makes statistical analysis more complex but has the advantages of facilitating the control selection (because there is no prior matching) and allowing the use of the same control population for other comparisons within the cohort. Under certain conditions, the case-cohort approach can be applied to a very large population (e.g., the inhabitants of a region).

Case-control study: This is an epidemiological design comparing previous exposure to a risk factor of interest (e.g., use of a specific health product) or the presence of a characteristic in a group of subjects presenting a given event (the *cases*) to that in a group not presenting this event (the *controls*) (see Chapter 3 for more information). The two groups may differ in size but, except for the presence of the event of interest, must be as similar as possible with respect to the main factors that could influence the probability of exposure to the risk factor(s). The comparability could theoretically be guaranteed by a random selection of cases and controls from the same source population but is generally attempted through either a priori matching and/or a posteriori adjustment or stratification, considering potential confounding variables. To obtain sufficient statistical power, it may be necessary to match each case to several controls, if the prevalence of exposure to the studied factor is low in the source population. The tested null hypothesis is that there is no association between exposure to the factor of interest and the occurrence of the event defining the cases. Under this hypothesis, we expect that the proportion exposed or the odds of exposure to this factor will be the same in the cases and controls. If this is not the case (i.e., the odds ratio differs significantly from 1), we conclude that there is an association, although not necessarily a causal one, between exposure and occurrence of the event. Thus, although a case-control study does not permit direct estimation of the risk, the value of the odds ratio quantifies the strength of the association between the exposure and the occurrence of the event. Moreover, in the absence of bias, and if the event of interest has a low probability of occurrence, the odds ratio is a good approximation of the relative risk linked to exposure (which could otherwise only be calculated with a cohort study). In pharmacoepidemiology, case-control studies are particularly useful in measuring the association between use of a health product and an adverse event of low probability and/or delayed occurrence. In such cases, a cohort study would require prolonged follow-up of a very large population.

Case-crossover study: This kind of study represents a form of epidemiological design to evaluate a possible association between an exposure and the occurrence of an event by comparing the number of cases arising within and outside a previously defined window of exposure, in a population whose exposure status changes over time. This method is applicable only under the following conditions:

- The follow-up of the population ensures the inclusion of all the cases arising during the study period.
- The exposure status is precisely known over the entire follow-up period.
- The exposure status of subjects changes during the follow-up.
- Under the hypothesis of the existence of a causal relationship between exposure and event and with reference to an occurrence mechanism, it is possible to define an exposure window during which an event induced by this exposure ought to occur.
- This time-window is short with respect to the duration of the follow-up of the cases.
- The a priori risk of the occurrence of the event is constant during each exposure window.

If these conditions are fulfilled, we compare the number of events occurring within the exposure window with the number of cases expected under the hypothesis of independence. This information is also discussed in Chapter 3.

Case definition: This word simply represents a set of criteria that permit the operational identification of the events investigated in a study. They should be precise, unambiguous, repeatable, reproducible, relevant, and pertinent to ensure the validity of measurements (e.g., an incidence rate). The case definition can be used to confirm the case status in case-control studies, to ascertain the outcomes in cohorts or clinical trials or in the framework of spontaneous reporting. Typically, the potential cases are assessed by an expert committee blind to exposure status using these criteria. *For example, thrombocytopenia can be defined as a platelet count below 100 g/L, in two measurements at least 1 week apart, with hemoglobin above 6.2 mmol/L and polynuclear neutrophils above 1.5 g/L in patients not treated with cytotoxic anticancer agents.* Such definition should be established prior to the beginning of the study.

Case-population study: This represents a case-cohort approach conducted within a cohort made up of the total population of a geographical area. The characteristics of cases occurring in the population (notably, their possible previous exposure to a given risk factor) are compared to those of the entire set of the subjects in this population (supposing that demographic, health, or drug-use statistics for the whole population are available). The validity of this approach assumes the existence of a surveillance system capable of identifying all the cases of an event within the population. The null hypothesis is that, in the absence of an association between exposure and event, the odds of exposure are identical among cases and the rest of the population, barring sampling variations. *Example: To discover whether the use of Xgeva increases the risk of hip fracture in the elderly, all the subjects over 65 years old residing in a given geographical area are studied. If, all the cases of hip fracture occurring in this region over a given period can be identified, and drug utilization in this population is known, it would be possible to compare the odds of exposure to the Xgeva in the cases with the odds in the entire population over 65 for the same period. If the odds are significantly greater than 1, it will be concluded that there is an association (causal or not causal) between the use of this Xgeva and the risk of hip fracture.*

Case report: This consists in the description of the clinical and laboratory data concerning the occurrence of an event in a single patient (useful for the passive surveillance of adverse drug reactions). The data elements pertaining to such regulatory transmission have been defined in the International Conference for Harmonization (ICH E2A).

Causality assessment method: As discussed in Chapters 2 and 3 this term represents a formalized procedure whose aim is to estimate the degree of plausibility of the conclusion that the use of a health product is the cause of an adverse event in a given patient.

Censoring: This word represents the absence of information, in a prospective study, about the fate of a certain number of subjects in the studied population. Censoring concerns subjects who had not presented the studied event by the time they were no longer followed because it is impossible to know whether or not they did later. For these subjects, the information is considered to be censored by the absence of a complete or longer follow-up. Censoring may be the result of various phenomena: loss to follow-up, accidental or natural death unrelated to the studied event, late inclusion of the subject, early termination of the study, and others. *For example, we are studying the 5-year recurrence rate among 500 subjects receiving a new anticancer treatment (Zytiga for the treatment of prostate cancer); 220 subjects were still alive and without recurrence at the end of 5 years, 148 had a recurrence during the follow-up, and 132 were not followed for the planned 5 years but had not presented a recurrence during the course of their incomplete follow-up. In this case it is impossible to know whether or not subjects in the last group would have presented a recurrence during the remaining part of the 5-year interval.* By extension, censoring may also apply to lack of information about a parameter of interest before a given date. *For example, in a database study of the effects of a treatment (Rituxan) among* *patients suffering from rheumatoid arthritis, it is not known whether the patients treated with Rituxan were, or were not, treated with a drug B (Celebrex) before the beginning of the information gathering. This information is said to be censored for these subjects.* It may or may not be appropriate to consider the available part of censored information in the final analysis, depending on the situation.

Chance: This word consists in the possibility of a random occurrence. Chance can be quantified with a probability, whether arbitrarily fixed or estimated by a calculation. *Example: A probability of .7 means that an event has 70 chances over 100 of occurring during a given period of time.*

Clinical trial: This general term represents any investigation in human subjects intended to discover or verify the clinical, pharmacological, and/or other pharmacodynamic effects of an investigational product(s), and/or to identify any adverse reactions to an investigational product(s), and/or to study the absorption, distribution, metabolism, and excretion (pharmacokinetic) of an investigational product(s) with the object of ascertaining its safety and/or efficacy to be able to calculate a risk/benefit ratio. The terms "clinical trial" and "clinical study" are synonymous (see ICH E6 on Good Clinical Practice for further information).

Closed population: This word usage in biostatistics studies consists in a population (e.g., a cohort) whose members are not renewed during the study period. Its size thus tends to decrease over time (due to deaths, loss to follow-up, and others) and the average age of its participants tends to increase. The definition does not necessarily imply that all subjects are included at the same time but that there is no recruitment once the predefined sample size has been reached. In this sense, "closed" is often synonymous with "fixed," although the latter may be used in other contexts.

Cluster, clustering: This represents the higher than expected incidence of an event in a given region (spatial cluster or place cluster), during a given period (temporal cluster or time cluster) or both (space–time or time–place cluster).

Cohort: This important word in epidemiological studies consists in a group of subjects selected according to one or more common characteristic(s) and followed over time to identify, describe, or quantify an event. In pharmacoepidemiology, the subjects are usually identified according to their exposure to a drug (or class of drugs), and the event or outcome exposure of interest can be a therapeutic effect, an adverse effect, a behavior, or any other criterion relevant to the evaluation of the effects induced by the exposure. The term "cohort" does not imply a given design or sample size: the study can include a small or large sample, with or without a control group (the control group being formed randomly or nonrandomly, and with or without matching). In pharmacovigilance, the term "cohort study" most often refers to a post-marketing observational study, an observational study without a control group, which is carried out following the market authorization of a health product.

Most postmarketing observational studies are multipurpose studies; they should comply with regulatory guidelines for postmarketing studies. The population of a cohort is said to be "fixed" if new subjects are not included during the study, and "dynamic" if they are. The length of follow-up can be identical for all the members of the cohort (cohort with fixed follow-up) or variable. In the latter case, a calculation using incidence density can be useful to take into account the varying contribution of individual subjects to the total follow-up time.

Cohort effect, generation effect: This represents the difference(s) observed between two or more groups of individuals with respect to state of health (e.g., the incidence rate of a disease) or exposure status, linked to the fact that these individuals were not born during the same period (i.e., do not belong to the same generation). A cohort effect thus reflects the influence of changes over time on the population containing the groups (e.g., in environment, quality of life, state of hygiene, the health-care system, etc.). *For example, the rate of valvulopathy is higher in the cohort of individuals born between 1940 and 1950 than in that of individuals born between 1960 and 1970. We know that the primary cause of valvulopathy is rheumatic heart disease during a childhood streptococcal infection, and that the treatment of childhood tonsillitis with penicillin was much more systematic after 1960.* Similarly, the term "cohort effect" is used to demonstrate the change in the risk of occurrence of an event during a prolonged follow-up of a nonrenewed population.

Cohort study, follow-up study, prospective study: This is a kind of epidemiological study based on the follow-up of one or more cohort(s). The objective of following a single cohort is generally to describe or quantify a phenomenon (i.e., a descriptive study). Comparative analysis of two or more cohorts seeks to explain the mechanism of or attribute a cause to the occurrence of an event.

Completeness of data, consistency of data: In pharmacovigilance, this term represents the informative value of collected data. This depends on the quantity and quality (in terms of relevance and validity) of the data available. *For example, an incompleteness of data can preclude imputability analyses, as it is impossible or even hazardous to investigate a causal association between the use of a health product and the occurrence of an event in poorly documented cases.* This is a kind of weakness that can interfere with the passive surveillance of adverse drug reactions in pharmacovigilance activities.

Compliance: This term is very useful for the success of a study and represents the respect, by a patient, of the directions for use of a therapy (medicinal or otherwise) he or she is meant to obey. These are generally conveyed by the health-care providers giving the prescription, although some authors extend the definition to include recommendations made by the pharmacist dispensing the health-care product or those provided in the package insert or the Canadian product monograph, for example. A patient is said to be *compliant* if his or her behavior does not vary significantly from what is expected, and *noncompliant* if this is not the case. Although at times difficult to assess, awareness of a subject's compliance is fundamental to characterizing the exposure of a population and the interpretation of some therapeutic failures or adverse events.

Concurrent: This term is used to indicate a prospective, retrospective, or cross-sectional approach to investigate events occurring after the beginning of the study. The term "historical," on the other hand, indicates an approach using previously recorded data. The term "prospective" should not be used as a synonym for concurrent, being reserved to indicate a study plan based on the follow-up of a population.

Conditional probability: This consist in a probability whose value is modified according to whether a given fact or result is taken into account. *Example: What is the probability that the subject uses benzodiazepines, knowing that he or she is (or is not) being treated with antidepressants?* The theory of conditional probabilities was formalized by the Bayes' theorem, in which the *prior probability* (estimated before analysis of a file, case, or situation) is multiplied by one or more *likelihood ratio(s)* calculated from the available data.

Confidence: This term represents the probability that an estimate, statement, or conclusion reflects the reality. In the strictest sense, this certainty corresponds to a confidence level of 100%. A confidence level of 95% means that a conclusion has 95 chances in 100 of being correct, or that we accept, at the most, a 5% risk of error.

Confidence interval: This term is particularly useful in pharmacoepidemiologic studies and consists in measuring the value of a parameter in a sample, the set of values having a given probability (called confidence) of including the real but unknown value (which could be measured in the whole population from which the sample was drawn). This calculation is inferential in that one concludes, at a fixed confidence level, that the real value of the parameter lies between the two limits of the interval. A confidence interval is called two-sided or two-tailed if both limits have been calculated [e.g., (0.025, 0.17)] and one-sided or one-tailed if only one limit has been calculated, the other being fixed a priori [e.g., (0, 0.07) or (12.9)]. *Example: If four cases of an event have been observed during the follow-up of 1800 persons treated with a drug, the two-sided 95% confidence interval calculated with the Poisson distribution around the observed proportion, 4/1800 or 0.002, lies between 0.0006 and 0.006. This means that the real risk of presenting this event during treatment has 95 chances in 100 of being between 6 and 60 per 10,000.* (See text of Chapter 3 to have further concrete examples of the use of confidence interval.)

Confounding, confounding variable, confounder: This important term used in epidemiological studies concerns the systematic error resulting from the fact that a secondary variable (called the *confounder* or *confounding variable*) is linked both to the exposure and to the event of interest, which can wholly or partially explain their association found in an epidemiological study. For instance, we falsely conclude to a direct and causal association between *E* (exposure) and *D* (disease) when they are in fact linked by the intermediate third variable acting as a confounder, *C*. The failure of taking possible confounding variables into account can strongly bias the estimate of the association between the exposure and the event. *Example: In the 1990s, a study found a strong association between use of oral contraceptives and risk of malignant melanoma. It subsequently became evident that the women who used oral contraceptives, being younger, exposed themselves to the sun more often than nonusers. An adjustment for duration of sun exposure substantially decreased the value of the odds ratio quantifying the strength of the association between oral contraceptives and malignant melanoma. Sun exposure, linked both to the probability of oral contraceptive use and the occurrence of malignant melanoma, acted as a confounder in this study.* Only the use of a controlled trial with randomization allows complete control of confounding, by distributing the known and the unknown potential confounders in a balanced manner between the groups. In observational epidemiology we can aspire to control the principal factors suspected to be confounders with matching or adjustment. (Chapter 3 also provides an excellent discussion about the impacts of confounders.)

Confounding by indication, prescription bias, prescription channeling: This particular instance of confounding, leading to a distorted estimate of the association between the use of a health product and the occurrence of an event, because a given drug (or class of drugs) is preferentially prescribed to subjects who have, a priori, a higher or lower risk of presenting the event in question. *For example, a new nonsteroidal antiinflammatory presented as being better tolerated by the digestive system could be the cause of a particularly high number of gastrointestinal hemorrhages if it is preferentially prescribed to subjects at risk for this outcome. On the other hand, a health product correctly or incorrectly reputed to be poorly tolerated could be preferentially prescribed to subjects with a lower risk of presenting this effect (gastrointestinal hemorrhages).*

Confounding ratio: This is a relevant term used in epidemiologic study that consist in the ratio of the crude (unadjusted) value of a relative risk or an odds ratio to the value of this parameter after adjustment by a factor considered to be a confounder. The value of this ratio quantifies the extent of the confounding by the factor (a ratio of 1 indicating the absence of confounding). *Example: In a cohort study comparing the risk of venous thrombosis associated with two types of oral contraceptives has resulted in a relative risk estimate of 4.2. After the adjustment for the duration of contraception, the value of this relative risk is 1.7. The confounding ratio,* *equal to 4.2/1.7 = 2.5, indicates that the duration of the contraception acts as a confounder in this study.*

Continuity correction: This represents a correction applied to a statistic test when a continuous probability distribution is used to approximate a discrete distribution (e.g., when a test based on the normal or Chi-square distributions is used to compare the distribution of a characteristic or number of events in two small samples). A continuity correction tends to make the test more conservative by decreasing the probability of falsely rejecting the tested null hypothesis. The continuity corrections always make shift, and it is preferable to use a test based on the appropriate probability distribution (e.g., Fisher's exact test, to compare a distribution when one or more number(s) are small).

Contributing factor: This is a relevant word used to designate a factor whose presence is likely to increase the probability of the occurrence of an adverse event. This term is most often used in pharmacovigilance. In epidemiology, the terms "risk factor" or "effect modifier" are generally preferred.

Control, control group: This represents a subject, or group of subjects, used as a reference in a comparison trial. Ideally, the controls are drawn from the same reference population as the cases under study and differ from the latter only with respect to the absence of the factor whose influence is being measured.

Controlled trial, comparative trial: This important term in pharmacoepidemiology represents a prospective clinical trial in which a health product or therapeutic strategy is compared to a reference (control) (see text in Chapter 3). The object of the comparison can be a therapeutic efficacy, a tolerance, or any other criterion (pharmacokinetic parameters, cost, quality of life, etc.). The reference used can be an inert substance (placebo) or another strategy—medicinal or nonmedicinal—recognized as being efficacious. The method may employ a parallel group or a crossover strategy; in either case, the allocation of treatments may be randomized. Similarly, the nature of this allocation may be unknown to the patient, the investigator, or both (single-blind, double-blind).

Cost–benefit study, cost–benefit analysis, cost–benefit: This is another kind of study aimed at comparing the costs and the consequences of a therapeutic strategy, expressed in monetary terms. *Example: The cost of a vaccination campaign can be compared with the cost of treating the cases of the disease, which would be or were avoided by the vaccination.*

Cost-effectiveness study: This is a kind of study aimed at linking the cost of a strategy to one or more indicator(s) of effectiveness expressed in physical and not monetary terms. The cost is expressed in units of result (e.g., cost per year of life gained, cost per complication avoided, etc.). The term "cost-effectiveness" can be considered a synonym of efficiency.

Crossover trial, crossover study: This is a kind of controlled study where the exposure status of the subjects changes over time; each subject being successively exposed and then not exposed (or the reverse) becomes his or her own control (see text in Chapter 3). The change of status can be imposed by the protocol (i.e., a crossover trial) or observed without intervention (i.e., an observational crossover study). In a clinical crossover trial, the state of the subjects is compared under two treatments, A and B, possibly repeated and sometimes separated by a period without treatment (*washout period*). It is preferable to randomly allocate the treatment to minimize the effect to the natural evolution of the studied phenomena (e.g., spontaneous improvement or worsening of the illness, influence of climate or season, etc.), or a carryover effect from one treatment to the other. Crossover studies are also widely used in pharmacoepidemiology.

Cross-sectional study, prevalence study: This term has already been explained in the text and represents the study in which the prevalence of a variable (e.g., exposure, an event, a disease) is measured in a population at a given moment; this can also be termed a prevalence study. In pharmacoepidemiology, cross-sectional studies can be used to measure, for example:

- The prevalence of a disease or an event in a population.
- The prevalence of exposure to a risk factor such as the use of a health product.

Example: A study consists of interviewing 2400 people chosen at random from a list on a given day; 32 of them used a given health product on this day. The prevalence of use of the health product in this region is 1.3%. In a cross-sectional study there is, by definition, neither follow-up nor analysis of past events. It is nevertheless possible to study the potential association between an event and a characteristic (e.g., an exposure); however, the absence of temporal analysis of the exposure/event relationship can lead to errors in interpretation, such as *reverse causality bias. For example, in a cross-sectional study of a population, we find greater use of aspirin in hypertensive subjects than in those with normal blood pressure. This difference being statistically significant after adjustment for age and gender, we conclude that aspirin use is a risk factor for arterial hypertension. In fact, the use of aspirin by hypertensives can be partly explained by preventive use, as stroke can be induced by systemic hypertension. An approach based on the analysis of the chronological exposure/event sequence would have prevented this interpretative error.*

Database: This is an important tool for the active surveillance of adverse drug reactions and represents a set of logically connected data or files accessible with specialized software. The data can be classified according to geographical origin (*population database*), by exposure to a risk factor (e.g., the subjects treated with a given health product), by the presence of a disease, and others. Large population databases (such as the Canada Vigilance or the WHO databases) that gather information on many millions of people are very useful sources of observational data for pharmacoepidemiology studies. See Chapter 2 for more information and Chapter 4 presents concrete example on the use of databases.

Dependence, pharmacodependence: This represents the totality of behavioral, cognitive, and physiological phenomena, of varying intensity, in which the use of one or more psychoactive substance(s) becomes a high priority. The essential characteristics are the obsessive desire to procure and to take the causal substance and a constant pursuit for obtaining it. The determining factors of dependence and the ensuing problems may be biological, psychological, or social. The state of dependence is not necessarily harmful by itself but may result in self-administration of the causal substance in doses producing physical or behavioral effects that constitute social and public health problems. The term "pharmacodependence" is more and more often being replaced by "dependence."

Dependent variable: This is an important word to designate a variable whose value is modified by the presence or the value of another variable.

Descriptive study: This is another important term in pharmacoepidemiology to designate any epidemiological study whose goal is to identify a phenomenon, describe it, measure its frequency, and/or study its development and distribution in different subgroups of a population, but not to determine its cause or determinants. Even though the distinction between a descriptive study and an aetiologic study may be somewhat artificial, descriptive studies generally use a prospective approach (cohort study), without a comparison group.

Design, research design: This is a plan, a protocol, a strategy, or a scheme for a study.

Determinant: This is a factor that influences the probability of the occurrence of an event or disease, or the state of health of a population. This factor may act alone or in association with other factors; however, the term "determinant" (as opposed to *risk factor*) implies a causal association with the disease.

Diagnostic bias: This is an important term in pharmacoepidemiology studies that represents a selection bias in which a case has a different probability of being diagnosed according to whether he or she is exposed to a risk factor of interest or not. *Example: In a cohort study designed to assess the risk of PML associated with Rituxan, a physician might be inclined to seek this symptom more actively if he or she knows that the patient is treated by this drug.*

Directionality: This is the direction of reference to time in an epidemiological study (i.e., *prospective*, *retrospective*, or *cross-sectional*).

Discrete variable: This term simply concerns a variable that may only assume a certain number of integer values within its limits of variation (e.g., number of children per couple, number of episodes of an illness, etc.), unlike a continuous variable.

Drug, medication, medicine, medicinal product: This term consists in any substance or combination of substances that may be administered to human beings or animals with a view to making a medical diagnosis or to restoring, correcting, or modifying a physiological function. This term thus applies not only to substances intended to treat a disease or symptom but also to vaccines, contrast media, and other agents administered for diagnostic purposes, intravenous solutions, blood products, oral contraceptives, and others.

Dynamic: This is an adjective designating a population whose composition changes during the follow-up period because some subjects have left it whereas others have joined the population. Thus, on any given date, the effective duration of follow-up or the time elapsed since the beginning of the exposure can differ to some extent for each member of the population. This term is also used to designate any event or variable whose nature or value changes over time.

Ecological: This term represents any study or analysis carried out not on one or more population(s) with individuals selected according to a protocol but on global population data (*aggregated data*), available at the regional or national level, and generally not collected for this purpose (see text). This approach is extremely useful because it allows rapid exploration of a large number of hypotheses without requiring the implementation of a specific data collection. However, the absence of information about the characteristics of individuals and the conditions of their possible exposure to the risk factor of interest makes this approach particularly subject to numerous biases and interpretative errors. *Example: In Nunavut, a research team observed an increase in mortality from syphilis proportional to the number of prescriptions of a new drug, using national statistics. This could have corresponded to a particular risk associated with the drug but also to an unrelated increase in the incidence of transmissible diseases in the province, leading to increased prescription of the drug.*

Effect, reaction: This term represents a modification of a previous state, which can reasonably be attributed to an exposure, particularly to a health product (e.g., *therapeutic effect, adverse reaction*). If the causal relationship with the exposure (the health product) is not established or at least strongly suspected, the term "event" should be used instead (because *effect* implies that the event was induced by the exposure).

Effectiveness, effective: This consists in the demonstration of the therapeutic effect of a health product under real conditions of prescription and use.

Efficacy, efficacious: This is a major term associated with the approbation of a new health product for marketing and represents the ability to produce the expected effect. A drug is qualified "efficacious" if it can induce a therapeutic effect. A distinction should be made between the terms "active" and "efficacious." The first most often applies to a substance or a health product that causes one or more pharmacodynamic effect(s) that may induce a therapeutic effect (e.g., an active principle, pharmacological activity). The term "efficacious" is applied to a health product whose therapeutic effect has been demonstrated under standardized or experimental conditions such as clinical trials. "Efficacy" differs from "effectiveness," the latter referring to the demonstration of a drug's therapeutic effect under real conditions of prescription and use, i.e., in postmarketing context.

Epidemiological study: This relevant term concerns the study whose objective is to describe the characteristics, behavior, or state of health of a population (i.e., a *descriptive study*), or to investigate the associations (causal or otherwise) that may exist within this population between a characteristic (e.g., the exposure to a risk factor) and the occurrence of an event (i.e., an *aetiologic study*). Three major types of epidemiological study can be described, according to the *directionality* of the analysis (see Chapter 3):

- *Prospective or cohort studies* in which a population is followed after the beginning of an exposure, to investigate how much this modifies the probability of the occurrence of an event (the causal inference being from exposure to event).
- *Retrospective studies* (e.g., case-control studies) in which an exposure is sought for the previous history of subjects having presented an event (the causal inference being from event to exposure).
- *Cross-sectional studies*, which analyze the state of health or the characteristics of a population at a given moment, with neither a follow-up nor an analysis of the past.

Epidemiology: This is the study of the relationships between diseases or any other biological phenomenon and various factors (e.g., lifestyle, environment or social setting, individual traits, etc.), which can influence their frequency, distribution, and evolution. Several somewhat arbitrary distinctions can be made:

- *Descriptive epidemiology* in which the objective is to describe a population (e.g., drug utilization studies),
- *Analytic epidemiology* in which the objective is to study the associations (causal or otherwise) that can exist, within a population, between the occurrence of an event and a given characteristic (e.g., exposure to a risk factor).

Equivalence: This represents a state that can be considered identical or differing at most by a negligible amount. Two therapeutic strategies can thus be considered equivalent if they induce—both qualitatively and quantitatively—the same effects. Equivalence may apply to both therapeutic and adverse effects. The term "bioequivalence" is used to indicate the fact that two health products induce the same active plasma concentrations in an organism during a period that covers the absorption and elimination phases, by which the identical (qualitative and quantitative) biological, pharmacological, and therapeutic effects may be expected. In this instance equivalence is defined by regulatory criteria. This term will be further explained in Chapter 4.

Estimation: This is a procedure consisting of determining, as precisely as possible, the unknown value of a parameter in a population, based on a measurement made on a sample taken from this population. Estimation is, by definition, an inferential procedure. The term "estimate" indicates the result of this procedure.

Event: This important term represents any phenomenon that can be observed or studied in a subject or population. In pharmacovigilance, "event" designates a desirable or undesirable manifestation without presuming that it is or not related to the use of a health product. This term is also used each time the numbers of cases occurring in two populations, of which one is not exposed, are compared; it would be incorrect to speak of an "effect" in a population that has not been exposed to a risk factor (such as the use of a health product).

Expected adverse drug reaction, expected adverse effect: This consists in a harmful and undesirable manifestation attributed to a health product, whose occurrence is apparently related to a known pharmacological property of the health product. The term "expected" implies that the knowledge of the pharmacological properties of a health product makes it possible to foresee such adverse events in a certain proportion of treated patients. *Examples: Kaliuresis with loop diuretics, prolonged bleeding time with aspirin.* To accept that this effect is the expression of a pharmacological property of the health product implies that it will be found in an appreciable proportion of treated patients, that it is generally dose-dependent and will be reproducible, in whole or part, in animals. In this sense, an expected adverse effect is synonymous with "side effect" and is sometimes also called a "Type A reaction." By extension and somewhat abusively, an expected adverse drug reaction is considered the same as a *labeled effect*. Indeed, the current international definition designates an expected adverse effect as a manifestation clearly mentioned in the Canadian product monograph, summary product characteristics, package insert, or investigator's brochure for a clinical trial.

Expected number: This represents that the number of cases of an event is expected to be observed in a given population during a given period. This is calculated by multiplying the number of surveyed units n in this population (e.g., number of subjects, number of risk periods, etc.) by the probability p of occurrence of the event for each unit considered. *Example: If the annual incidence of multiple sclerosis is 30 per million inhabitants, the expected number per month among 500,000 subjects (assuming that the incidence rate* *is constant) is (30/1,000,000) = 500,000 = 1/12 = 1.25*. The observed number of cases may differ more or less significantly from the expected number. This variability can be predicted by an adequate probability model. For example, the *prediction interval* constructed around the expected number of events defines the set of values for the number of cases with a given probability of being observed.

Experimental: Here we discuss about an adjective designating a strategy in which the researcher intentionally alters the natural course of events for the purposes of research. The classical experimental design consists of artificially creating two groups (e.g., by randomly allocating exposure) that are identical with respect to the variables that can influence the planned measurement and differ only in their exposure status. Under these strict conditions, any statistically significant difference observed between the two groups (not explained by sampling variation) can be attributed to the studied factor. In clinical research, these modifications are formalized in advance by a protocol. A typical experimental design is a Phase III clinical trial in which groups are made comparable by randomization.

Explanatory trial: Experimental controlled trial. This important term consists in an explanatory trial that compares (under standardized conditions) two or more randomly constituted groups, which are therefore deemed to differ only with respect to the status of the factor under study (see text in Chapter 3 for further explanation of this term). The explanatory trial is an undisputable reference for any etiologic analysis. It is used as much in clinical pharmacology (e.g., controlled trials with randomization) as in analytic epidemiology.

Exploratory study: This term represents a study in which the objective of the research is not precisely defined beforehand. The term "exploratory" may apply to studies that are perfectly scientifically justified when, for example, nothing is known about the effects of a new health product, or if the objective of the study is specifically to learn whether it would be appropriate to undertake a particular study or to refine its protocol (i.e., a *feasibility study*).

Exposed: This important term designs the subject or population presenting a precisely defined characteristic that may increase the probability of occurrence of an event or disease. This characteristic could be, for example, past or present contact with a pathogen (e.g., bacteria, virus, radiation, and others). In pharmacoepidemiology, the term "exposed" designates a patient treated by one or more health product(s) under conditions (such as dose or duration) that place him or her at risk for a given adverse effect. This term also applies to indirect exposure (e.g., exposure in utero or an infant's exposure to a drug via breast-feeding). The risk period does not necessarily correspond to the treatment period: for an effect with delayed onset (e.g., cancer), subjects are considered at risk (i.e., exposed) even though their treatment dates back several years. In other respects, not every treated subject is necessarily at risk of presenting the effect: if it cannot occur until after 3 months of treatment, subjects treated for 1 week are not at risk and should be considered nonexposed.

Exposed/not-exposed study: This term represents a prospective etiologic study design based on the follow-up and comparison of two populations, of which only one is exposed to the factor whose influence on the occurrence of an event under study. If exposure is determined by chance, an exposed/not-exposed study is the same as an explanatory or experimental-controlled clinical trial. With respect to observational pharmacoepidemiology, an exposed/not-exposed study is equivalent to a cohort study with a reference group.

False negative: This term designs the negative diagnostic test result in a subject who has the disease under study. By analogy, this term is also used when a surveillance method does not detect a case corresponding to the definition of the event of interest.

False positive: This term designs the positive diagnostic test result in a subject who does not have the disease under study. By analogy, this term is also used when a surveillance method detects a case that is not related to the event of interest, or wrongly attributes the occurrence of the event to the risk factor of interest (e.g., consumption of a particular health product).

Fixed: In pharmacoepidemiology, this term can describe:

- A population whose members are not renewed by the inclusion of new subjects (e.g., a *fixed cohort*).
- A follow-up period that is identical for all of the members of a population (i.e., a cohort with a fixed follow-up).

Follow-up: This consists in a prospective surveillance set up to identify the occurrence of an event in an individual or population. The term applies only when the surveillance method is effective and relevant to the event of interest.

Frequency: This represents the quantification of the total number of events in a population (i.e., *prevalence*) or only those cases occurring during the study period (i.e., *incidence*). The term is often used to designate relative frequency, that is, the number of cases of an event compared to the size of the study population and the duration of the follow-up. In this case, frequency is synonymous with prevalence or incidence rate.

General population: This represents a geographically defined population (e.g., the inhabitants of a city, region, or country). This population is usually heterogeneous and can include subjects having very different characteristics. A risk, incidence rate, or prevalence rate estimated in the general population can thus be very different from that which would be measured in an ad hoc reference group.

Generic drug: This term designs a drug (health product) that has the same qualitative and quantitative compositions in active ingredient(s) and the same pharmaceutical form, as the reference drug whose bioequivalence has been demonstrated by appropriate studies. The marketing of a generic drug is only possible after the end of the period of patent protection of the copied innovation (e.g., active principle, manufacturing process, form, new association, and others).

Gold standard test: This term represents in medicine and statistics, a test that is usually the diagnostic test or the benchmark that is the best available under reasonable conditions. Other times, gold standard is the most accurate test possible without restrictions. A hypothetical ideal "gold standard" test has a sensitivity of 100% with respect to the presence of the disease (it identifies all individuals with a well-defined disease process; it does not have any false-negative results) and a specificity of 100% (it does not falsely identify someone with a condition that does not have the condition; it does not have any false-positive results).

GRADE system: GRADE offers a system for rating the quality of evidence in systematic reviews and guidelines and grading strength of recommendations in guidelines. The system is designed for reviews and guidelines that examine alternative management strategies or interventions, which may include no intervention or current best management. The GRADE process begins with asking an explicit question, including specification of all important outcomes. After the evidence is collected and summarized, GRADE provides explicit criteria for rating the quality of evidence that includes study design, risk of bias, imprecision, inconsistency, indirectness, and magnitude of effect. Recommendations are characterized as strong or weak (alternative terms conditional or discretionary) according to the quality of the supporting evidence and the balance between desirable and undesirable consequences of the alternative management options. In the GRADE approach, randomized controlled trials (RCTs) start as high-quality evidence and observational studies as low-quality evidence supporting estimates of intervention effects. Ultimately, the quality of evidence for each outcome falls into one of four categories from high to very low. Guideline developers (but not systematic reviewers) then review all the information to make a final decision about which outcomes are critical and which are important and come to a final decision regarding the rating of overall quality of evidence. Guideline (but not systematic review) authors then consider the direction and strength of recommendation. The balance between desirable and undesirable outcomes and the application of patients' values and preferences determine the direction of the recommendation, and these factors, along with the quality of the evidence, determine the strength of the recommendation. Both direction and strength may be modified after taking into account the resource use implications of the alternative management strategies. Because most existing systematic reviews do not adequately address all relevant outcomes (many, for instance, are restricted to RCTs), the GRADE process may require relying on more than one systematic review.

Hazard function, risk function: This is the representation of the evolution of the probability of occurrence of an event as a function of time. Ideally, this evolution in risk is estimated from repeated measurements of the instantaneous incidence rate, carried out at regular and sufficiently close intervals in a population adequately followed over a period of time. For some researchers, a hazard or risk function also denotes a mathematical model allowing prediction of the instantaneous risk at a given time during the follow-up.

Hazard rate, attack rate: This represents the probability that a subject, as yet unaffected, will present the event of interest during a very short time interval, approaching zero. It is estimated from an instantaneous incidence rate.

Historical: This represents an adjective denoting a study that uses prerecorded data. The events of interest that have occurred prior to the implementation of the study are investigated, for example, using a database. In a *historical cohort study*, the subjects are followed beginning at a date in the past, toward the present, with the aim of finding events that may have occurred.

Historical cohort: This is a kind of cohort whose population is identified and followed-up based on prerecorded data, usually collected for other purposes (e.g., in a population database). A study based on a cohort of this type remains a prospective study insofar as the possible occurrence of an event after the beginning of the subjects' exposure to the risk factor of interest (even if the events occurred and were recorded prior to the implementation of the study) is investigated.

Hypothesis: This term designs the proposition accepted provisionally before being tested.

Iatrogenic: This term reflects a health problem induced by a health-care provider or medical treatment. "Iatrogenesis" covers all of the consequences of medical intervention that are proved to be, or may potentially be, harmful to health (e.g., diagnostic errors, maladapted prevention or prescription, complications of a therapeutic act). "Medication iatrogenesis" refers to all the consequences of medication (whether prescribed or used in self-medication) that are proved to be, or may potentially be, harmful to health. Its scope is therefore wider than that of expected or unexpected adverse effects alone because it also includes the confirmed ineffectiveness of a poorly adapted treatment, the effects induced by the context of the prescription (*nocebo effect*) and the creation of a state of dependence.

Imputability, attributability, case-by-case causality assessment: This represents the estimate of the possible causal link between a drug treatment and the occurrence of an adverse event in a given patient. The aim of imputability analysis is to determine the degree of plausibility of the assumption that a given health product caused the adverse effect presented by a patient. This assessment is thus strictly individual and does not refer to the potential danger of the health product in the absolute or the significance of the risk for a population. Various methods have been published or proposed to standardize the process of imputation and thereby reduce inter- and intra-observer variability. These are based either on algorithms (classic imputability methods) or on theories of conditional probabilities (e.g., Bayesian methods). The former are used more often in routine surveillance and make use of the sequential evaluation of a given number of criteria, allowing calculation of an imputability score.

Incidence: This term consists in the number of new cases of an event identified in a population over a given period of time (e.g., incident cases, annual incidence, incidence rate, and others). In everyday language, this term is frequently used to designate an incidence rate (e.g., an annual incidence of 3 per 1000).

Incidence rate: This term represents the number of new cases of an event occurring in a population during a given period, divided by the number of subjects at risk in the population. The incidence rate represents the speed of production of new cases in the population, per unit of time. It is the fundamental parameter for estimating the risk of an event or disease in a population, or for a subject or subgroup of this population. The number of cases appearing in the population can be compared to the number of subjects followed during the period of interest or to the sum of follow-up or exposure times of the subjects making up the population (*incidence density*). In pharmacoepidemiology the study population is usually an exposed population, due to treatment with a health product, but can also be an untreated population (e.g., a reference or general population). For an incidence rate, subjects having presented the event (constituting the numerator) are a subgroup of the total studied population (the denominator); each subject in the population theoretically has the same baseline probability of presenting the event. The subjects with abnormally low or zero probability of presenting the event (e.g., those treated for too short a period to be at risk, or subjects physiologically unable to present the event of interest) should not be included in the calculation of the denominator, neither should those who have not been surveyed in a manner that will guarantee the identification of the event of interest.

Independent variable: This is a kind of variable whose status or value affects that of another variable. For example, in a regression model, the value of a dependent variable is predicted by the value(s) of one or more independent (or explanatory) variable(s).

Inference: This represents the extrapolation of the results drawn from a measurement or an estimate made from a study sample to a larger population (usually, from which the sample was drawn).

Information bias, observational bias: This represents the distortion of the estimate of the association between a risk factor (e.g., use of a drug) and the occurrence of an adverse event, due to a systematic difference in the way information concerning the measured parameter is collected for the groups being compared. *Recall bias* and *interviewer bias* are types of information bias.

Intent-to-treat analysis: This is a kind of statistical analysis taking into account all evaluable patients included in a study of efficacy or tolerance. Contrary to analyses that retain only those subjects treated according to the protocol, an intent-to-treat analysis considers all subjects from the time of their inclusion in the study (e.g., once they have been allocated a randomization code in a parallel group trial), even if it turns out that a subject never took the prescribed treatment or modified its timing, dosage or duration, or if he or she left the study or is deceased. This type of approach has the great advantage of better reflecting the actual (or future) conditions of the doctor–patient and patient–medication relationships but tends to be more conservative (in diminishing the chances of observing a significant statistical difference between the groups, by increasing the intersubject variability). Intent-to-treat analyses can be used in clinical trials, both controlled and noncontrolled, and with or without blinding. The intent-to-treat approach may also be used in prospective (cohort) pharmacoepidemiological studies seeking to confirm an efficacy or to describe a risk or usage. For more information on this term, the readers may wish to consult the ICH-E9 on statistical principles for clinical trial at the section Resources for the Readers.

Interaction: In pharmacology, this represents the term designating a modification in effect (whether beneficial or adverse) obtained or expected from a health product, as the result of the concomitant use of another substance, whether medicinal or not or of the presence of another factor (e.g., age). An interaction is called "pharmacokinetic" if the second health product modifies—at whatever level—the pharmacokinetics, and thus the tissue concentration of the first (e.g., by accelerating or slowing down hepatic metabolism or renal elimination). In a "pharmacodynamic" interaction, the second health product does not affect the pharmacokinetics of the first product but interacts with its pharmacological action by inhibiting it (*antagonism*) or reinforcing it (*synergism*). In epidemiology, the term "interaction" (or *effect modification*) is used when the presence of a factor or the value of a variable modifies the effect produced by an exposure. This is the case when the strength of the association between an exposure and the occurrence of an event (e.g., quantified by the relative risk) is not the same in the presence or absence of another factor, called an "effect modifier." Observing an interaction sometimes allows identification of groups at risk. *Example: In a case-control study assessing the association between the use of a health product and the occurrence of acute pancreatitis, the odds ratio calculated for the entire group of subjects is 3. After stratification according to age, the odds ratio is 1.8 for subjects less than 65 years old and 5.2 for subjects 65 years and over. Age is thus a modifier of the risk; subjects over 65 years are a group at risk for this adverse effect. This example could also apply for alcohol consumption.*

Intermediate endpoint: This is a form of judgment criterion that predicts a priori a relevant clinical criterion, and it is used in place of the latter to temporarily assess the efficacy or tolerance of a therapeutic strategy (see ICH E9 Guidelines on Statistical Principles for Clinical trial). This means that the efficacy or tolerance will only be considered to have been truly assessed on the grounds of a study, or subsequent analysis, based on the relevant clinical criterion. On the other hand, a *surrogate endpoint* can be used instead of the relevant clinical criterion, once the validity of its predictive value has been established.

Intermediate factor: This is a kind of factor that does not constitute a cause in itself but that represents a crucial step in the exposure-to-effect chain. *For example, certain medications can result in liver injury, not by a direct effect, but by inducing low blood pressure causing hypoperfusion and thus hepatic anoxia; in this case, low blood pressure acts as an intermediate factor.*

Interventional, nonobservational: This represents an adjective characterizing a situation in which the normal course of events or the therapeutic relationship is voluntarily modified for the purposes of research, generally to create artificial situations or groups for the purposes of comparison under optimal conditions. This term is the antonym of "observational." An *experimental design* is the most interventional of the studies.

Interviewer bias: This is another important information bias in which the interviewer questions the subjects in a systematically different way according to whether they belong to one or the other of the groups being compared. This bias is classic in case-control studies when the interviewer knows the hypothesis being tested or is interested in its validation. He or she can, intentionally or not, question cases more precisely and insistently than controls regarding their exposure to the suspected risk factor. This term is also discussed in Chapter 3.

Intrinsic imputability: This term defines the analysis of the degree of responsibility of a health product for the occurrence of an adverse event in a given patient, not accounting for the degree of notoriety of this putative adverse effect. The analysis thus only takes into account the information drawn from the observed case.

Investigator: This defines the person or organization undertaking research according to a predefined protocol on behalf of, and usually at the request of, a *sponsor*. In multicentre researches involving many investigators in different sites, one of these investigators must be identified as the *main investigator*. For a legal definition of investigators, the reader may consult the Food and Drug Act and Regulations at the end of this book.

Latency period, latent period, latency: This represents the interval of time separating the beginning of exposure to a risk factor and the occurrence of an event. This term usually has a more restrictive meaning than "onset delay" in that it tends to imply a causal relationship between exposure and event. Indeed, "latency" designates the quiescent character of a process set off by exposure but appearing only much later, such as for cancer.

Longitudinal study: This is a somewhat ambiguous term used to define any study based on the follow-up of one or more group(s) of subjects. A longitudinal study may be considered a synonym for a *prospective study*, and, according to some researchers, for a cohort study. In practice, the term "longitudinal" is often used for descriptive studies based on the observation of a single cohort. Lastly, according to other authors, the term "longitudinal" may indicate any prospective or retrospective study in which, contrary to cross-sectional studies, a phenomenon is studied or a possible association between exposure and illness is investigated over a sufficiently long period of time.

Lost to follow-up: In a prospective study (e.g., a clinical trial or cohort study), the subjects have not been followed for the full extent of the planned term because there is no knowledge of outcome beyond a certain date for unknown reasons. In the strictest sense, it is also advisable to consider as lost to follow-up all subjects for whom information about their subsequent fate is available, but where the exhaustiveness and reliability of this information do not correspond to the quality criteria stated in the protocol. The lost to follow-up can certainly influence the validity of a clinical trial and therefore should be avoided as much as possible.

Matching: This procedure consists in rendering two groups (e.g., an exposed group and a reference group in a cohort study or a diseased group and a nondiseased group in a case-control study) as comparable as possible with respect to the distribution of certain variables capable of biasing the results of the proposed statistical analysis by acting as confounders. Matching consists of selecting, for each subject included in a study, one or several controls comparable with respect to the match variable(s). *Example: If in a case-control study we think that age could be a confounder (by being linked to both the disease that defines a case and the probability of exposure to the factor of interest), the two groups (cases and controls) should be rendered comparable with respect to age distribution. This may be achieved by selecting one or more control(s) for each recruited case of the same age as the case.* Matching only concerns known prognostic variables and cannot achieve the effectiveness of randomization. The latter is the only method capable of ensuring that known and unknown prognostic variables will be equally distributed among the groups being compared. Matching on a variable makes it impossible to study the effect of this variable on the studied outcome.

MedDRA: This defines the abbreviation for Medical Dictionary for Drug Regulatory Activities. This represents standardized international medical terminology selected and developed by the International Conference on Harmonisation (ICH). This thesaurus has thereby become officially adopted by most regulatory authorities. It includes all the terms from the previous adverse reaction terminologies (WHOART and COSTART) and a number of terms from the International Classification of Diseases (ICD). It also includes terms for medical or surgical procedures and for life events.

Metaanalysis: This is a statistical method in which the results of several trials or studies devoted to the same topic are combined, with the goal of obtaining greater statistical power or more accurate estimates. Metaanalysis has been most frequently applied to clinical trials (most notably, within the Cochrane Collaboration), but can be useful in pharmacoepidemiology (in cohort or case-control studies) to obtain, for example, a more accurate estimate of a relative risk or an odds ratio. Metaanalysis has, however, a number of significant limits linked to the difficulty in accessing the data sources of the studies, the validity of the data, and the fact that an unknown number of studies on the subject of interest may not have been published. This term is also discussed in Chapter 3.

Misuse: It is when the prescription or use of a health product that does not conform to the approved recommendations. Misuse is thus the opposite of "*proper use*," and, contrary to "*abuse*," may concern the prescriber as well as the user.

Model, modeling: This represents a simplified representation of a generally complex process or system. In this way, research on new drugs often leads to trials with *animal models* that are supposed to faithfully represent the human disease to some degree. The term "model" is also given to mathematical formula used to predict the probability of appearance of a disease or event based on the value of different variables (e.g., logistic model, Cox model).

Multicentre: This constitutes research (e.g., a study or trial) carried out at different sites by more than one investigator, but following the same protocol. This kind of study is often linked to Phase III studies (or pivotal studies).

NDA: This is the acronym for "new drug approval."

Negative predictive value: This represents the probability that a subject for whom a diagnostic test is negative is not diseased. The negative predictive value is calculated by dividing the number of *true negatives* (d) by the total number of times the test results are negative ($c + d$) (see the contingency table below):

	Diseased	Nondiseased	
Positive test	a	b	$a+b$
Negative test	c	d	$c+d$

Nested case-control, nested case-control design, nested case-control study: A case-control study is carried out within the population of a cohort, whether constructed for this purpose or not (see text in Chapter 3). All the subjects in the cohort having presented the event of interest during the follow-up (the *cases*) are compared, regarding exposure to the studied risk factor, with subjects in the cohort not having presented this event (the *controls*) with possible matching or adjustment. As opposed to classical case-control studies, absolute risk can be estimated.

Network: This represents a group of geographically distinct entities, persons, or structures collaborating on a common objective. In pharmacovigilance or pharmacoepidemiology, the term can designate a group of clearly identified, voluntary observers (physicians or pharmacists) regularly participating in a project coordinated by a single organization. The aim could be to identify or quantify a risk, or to describe the prescription or use of one or more health product(s).

Noncontrolled study, noncontrolled trial: This is a kind of study in which the value of a measurement is compared neither to a measurement taken from another sample nor to a reference value, known or fixed in advance. A noncontrolled strategy is frequently used in descriptive epidemiology to measure the frequency of a phenomenon, to describe it, or study its evolution with a longitudinal study. The terms "*open study*" and "*open trial*" have the same signification but can lead to confusion by implying that the sample population changes during the study period (the term "*open population*" often being used in epidemiology as a synonym for *dynamic population*).

Normal care relationship: This represents a therapeutic relationship in which contact with the patient, choice of treatment, expected benefit, incurred risks, and surveillance methods are neither modified nor organized by an external intervention. The health-care providers takes only the interests of the patient into account and not those of a third party interested in the results of a study, e.g., a sponsor; he or she is guided by the present state of medical knowledge and the recommendations of the scientific community or health authorities. The maintenance of the normal care relationship between the physician-researcher and the patient defines the conditions of an observational study.

Normal distribution, normal law, Gaussian distribution: The normal distribution is the probability distribution used most often for statistical tests and calculations (e.g., calculations of confidence intervals, comparisons of means, calculations of sample sizes, and others). The validity of these calculations and the resulting inferences requires, however, that the variable under consideration is distributed according to the normal law in the studied population. In the case of an approximation (e.g., of the binomial distribution by the normal distribution), it is advisable to verify the validity of this approximation (i.e., if the sample size is sufficiently large and the expected number of events is not too small).

Notoriety bias: This consists in a selection bias in which a case has a greater chance of being reported if the subject is exposed to the studied factor known to cause, thought to cause, or likely to cause the event of interest (see Chapter 3 for more information). *Example: This bias is classic in case-control studies of digestive tract bleeding. A health-care provider could be inclined to preferentially report cases for which exposure to a nonsteroidal antiinflammatory drug has been noted.*

Null hypothesis, test hypothesis: This important term in biostatistics represents a tested hypothesis that may possibly be rejected at the end of a study or calculation, in favor of another, called the *alternative hypothesis*. Both hypotheses should be clearly stated a priori. Type I error consists of wrongly rejecting the null hypothesis when it is true. Type II error consists of not rejecting the null hypothesis when it is false.

Observational study, nonexperimental study: This represents an approach in which the researcher merely observes a population or phenomenon without interfering in any way with the natural course of events (see text of Chapter 3 for more information). In this way, "observational" is equivalent to the term "*noninterventional*" used by some researchers. In clinical pharmacology, pharmacovigilance, and pharmacoepidemiology, a study can be described as "*observational*" if all aspects (e.g., allocation and length of treatment, surveillance method, risk incurred, and others) are carried out as if no study existed. The main value of such studies is that they are based on real-life situations (postmarketing setting) to describe them most faithfully. However, the absence of an experimental design increases the possibility of bias (notably confounding) and makes causal analysis difficult.

Odds: This represents the probability that an event will occur divided by the probability that it will not occur: *Odds = probability/1 − probability. Example: If 31 of 120 subjects have been exposed to a health product, the exposure odds of the health product for this population is 31/(120 − 31) = 0.35.*

Odds ratio: This important term in pharmacoepidemiology represents the ratio of two odds, each being the ratio of one probability to its complementary probability. The odds ratio is used often in epidemiology and pharmacoepidemiology, for three main following reasons:

- Unlike the relative risk, it can be calculated equally well in a prospective (cohort) study and in a retrospective (case-control) study.
- It has mathematical properties that permit analysis by common models, such as the logistic model.
- When the probability of occurrence of the event (the risk) is low, the odds ratio is practically equal to the relative risk, and thus constitutes a satisfactory or even very good approximation of the latter (see text in Chapter 3 for more information).

In a case-control study, we calculate the ratio of the odds of exposure to the factor of interest in the cases and controls:

	Cases	Controls
Exposed	*a*	*b*
Nonexposed	*c*	*d*

$OR = (a/c)/(b/d) = \mathrm{a} \times \mathrm{d/b} \times \mathrm{c}.$

One-sided test, one-tailed test: This is a statistical test in which the rejection area of the null hypothesis lies on only one side of this hypothesis. The prior choice of a one-sided test, rather than a two-sided one, generally allows a reduction in the sample size required to guarantee a given probability (power) of rejecting the null hypothesis when it is false.

Onset delay, time to onset: This represents the interval of time separating the beginning of exposure to a risk factor (e.g., treatment by a health product) and the occurrence of a phenomenon (e.g., an adverse event). Unlike the term "*latency period*," onset delay may be used even in the absence of an association between the two episodes and is a particularly useful term in the absence of a causal association.

Open study, open trial: According to different authors, *open study* has different meanings as follows:

- A *noncontrolled*, noncomparative study.
- A study based on a *dynamic*, i.e., renewed, sample.
- A nonblinded, controlled or noncontrolled, study.

Outcome: This is an expected or a measured result of exposure to a causal factor or of a therapeutic intervention.

Per protocol analysis: This is a kind of statistical principle that is based on patients having strictly conformed to the protocol in a study of efficacy or tolerance. This approach is preferably used in explanatory trials. For more information about this, the readers may wish to consult the ICH-E9 guidelines.

Peri-approval study, peri-approval trial: This is a kind of study or trial conducted immediately before or after drug approval is obtained with the aim of completing Phase III clinical trials, particularly with respect to tolerance. Such investigations almost always take the form of cohort studies. This concept is relevant for maintaining a positive product life cycle in terms of maintenance of the safety.

Personal therapeutic benefit: This represents a possible benefit to the health or well-being of a patient expected due to his or her participation in a biomedical research. Biomedical research (e.g., a clinical trial) can accordingly be described as being with or without personal therapeutic benefit. Research is generally said to have personal therapeutic benefit if at least some of the participating subjects can expect a benefit to their state of health or well-being. Thus, a blinded, randomized trial that compares the efficacy of a health product with that of a placebo may be deemed to have a personal therapeutic benefit even though, by definition, some of the patients in the trial, unknown in advance, will not receive the active treatment.

Person-time: This represents the sum of the follow-up times of each of the members of a population, generally used as the denominator of an incidence rate. This unit is particularly useful when the follow-up duration differs between subjects. It can be expressed in person-years, person-months, person-weeks, or person-days. When using data from spontaneous reporting in pharmacovigilance, it is customary to consider the duration of treatment, roughly estimated from sales data, rather than that of follow-up, and speak in terms of treatment-days (days of treatment), treatment-months (months of treatment), or treatment-years (years of treatment). *For example: 12 cases per 100,000 treatment-months means that, for the period and region of interest, 12 cases of an event were reported for a cumulative duration of drug treatment of 100,000 months. This conveys no information regarding the duration of each individual treatment: 100,000 treatment-months could correspond to 100,000 subjects treated for 1 month, 3.04 million subjects treated for 1 day, or 8333 subjects treated for 1 year; it is most likely that the treatment durations varied from subject to subject.*

Pharmacodynamic: This term is relative to the activity of a health product. The objective of the field of *pharmacodynamics* is to describe, quantify, and explain the set of effects induced by a drug in a living organism.

Pharmacodynamic effect: This represents an organic or biological, quantifiable, reproducible, and usually dose-dependent manifestation related to the administration of a health product to a living organism. The observation of a pharmacodynamic effect does not necessarily imply the existence of a therapeutic effect.

Pharmacoeconomics: This important type of epidemiological study concerns the evaluation of the medicoeconomic consequences attributable to the use of a health product. This assessment can be made before placing a health product on the market (predictive studies) or afterward, possibly including comparison with another strategy. The assessment may make use of predictive models, explanatory or pragmatic clinical trials, or observational studies.

Pharmacogenetics: This term designs the study of the variation of the effects or pharmacokinetics of a health product as a result of the genetic characteristics of a living organism. Because the majority of the sites of action and transformation of health products are genetically determined, a polymorphism may cause variations between individuals in the metabolism of, or response to, a given health product. *Example: In cancer or other diseases they are patients that are responding to specific health products because they possess a specific kind or receptor, but for those without this receptory, the response to treatment is considerably less. The pharmacogenetics is a step toward personalized medicine.*

Pharmacokinetics: This kind of study permits to determine the qualitative and the quantitative aspects of the fate of a health product within a living organism (human or animal). The harmacokinetics is concerned with the evolution of concentrations of a health product and its possible metabolites in the blood and certain biological tissues after or during the administration.

Pharmacology: This represents the study of interactions between drugs and living organisms. The term "*interaction*" should be understood to encompass the influence of a drug on a living organism (*pharmacodynamics*, *therapeutic effect*) and that of a living organism on a health product (*pharmacokinetics, metabolism*). *Clinical pharmacology* is concerned with the fate and effects of health product in human beings.

Phase I clinical trial: This is the first trial with a new active ingredient in humans. This type of trial is usually conducted on healthy volunteers, and its purpose is to assess tolerance as a function of dose and to carry out the first studies of clinical pharmacokinetics.

Phase II clinical trial: This represents a therapeutic pilot study designed to demonstrate efficacy and to assess short-term safety of an active ingredient in patients suffering from a disease or condition for which this active ingredient is intended. This type of trial is performed on a limited number of subjects and often, at the end of this phase, with a comparative protocol (e.g., against a placebo or a known comparator). Phase II trials are also used to determine the appropriate doses, dosages, and regimens and, if possible, to clarify the dose–response relationship, to provide an optimal basis for the design of therapeutic trials with a greater number of subjects. A distinction is sometimes made between Phase II trials, which characterize the pharmacodynamic effects of health products and study tolerance, and Phase II trials, focused on studying therapeutic activity as a function of dose.

Phase III clinical trial or pivotal trial: This is a type of trial involving larger and, if possible, more diversified groups of patients than those involved in Phases I or II to determine the short- and long-term risk/benefit ratio and to assess the overall and relative therapeutic value of one or more formulation(s) of an active ingredient. These trials permit the investigation of the type and profile of the most frequent adverse effects, as well as the clinically relevant drug interactions and the influence of factors such as age on the results. The trial protocol will preferably be randomized and double-blind, but other designs may be acceptable, especially for long-term safety studies. Generally, the conditions of a Phase III trial should be as close as possible to the normal conditions of use.

Phase IV: This term designs all studies or trials of a health product conducted after its marketing approval, and under the conditions (e.g., indication, dose, duration, and others) specified by this approval. The term "Phase IV," unlike Phases I, II, and III, does not imply a particular method or objective but refers to an administrative situation, namely the postapproval period.

Phase IV trial, Phase IV study: This is an important tool used in postmarketing and represents a trial or study of a health product conducted on the basis of the information (indications, dose, etc.) contained in the Canadian product monograph, for example. They can be useful for pharmacovigilance purposes or to assess the therapeutic utility or the cost of a strategy. Although prevailing conditions should be taken into account, Phase IV trials must be conducted with the same methodological rigor as in premarketing clinical trials and, at the very least, include a precise protocol. From a regulatory viewpoint, all postapproval trials designed to obtain an extension of the approval (e.g., for a new indication, new dosage, etc.) are Phase II or Phase III trials.

Placebo: This represents the substance or the pharmaceutical preparation or any other treatment presented as being therapeutically efficacious when it is in fact devoid of intrinsic activity but not necessarily of therapeutic effect. Such a substance can cause an improvement in the state of health or well-being of a patient (*placebo effect*) or provoke an adverse event (*nocebo effect*). When it is possible, the use of a placebo in one of the groups in a clinical trial (called a *placebo group*) allows estimation of the significance of the effects induced by the prescription, the prescription environment, or the simple fact of participation in a clinical study; an optimal reference is thus obtained for the quantification of the studied drug's effects.

Placebo effect: This represents a modification to the state of health or well-being of a subject not explained by a pharmacological property of a health product but apparently related to the psychological context surrounding its prescription, its environment, or the patient's confidence in the efficacy of the health product. This effect can also be observed with nonmedical treatments.

Point prevalence: This is the number of prevalent cases found in a given population during a very short time interval approaching zero.

Population-time: This is the sum of follow-up or exposure times for a population. This term is sometimes used to designate the amount of person-time used to calculate an incidence rate.

Positive predictive value: This is the probability that a subject for whom a diagnostic test is positive is diseased. The *positive predictive value* is calculated by dividing the number of *true positives* (a) by the number of times the test results are positive ($a + b$) (see contingency table below):

	Diseased	**Nondiseased**
Positive test	a	b
Negative test	c	d
	$a+c$	$b+d$

***Post hoc* analysis:** This is an analysis that was not anticipated or described before data collection. This kind of analysis can be performed on request based on concerns seen or make aware by a regulatory agency. This type of analysis is supported by the rule C.01.016 from the Food and Drug Regulations in Canada (see text in Chapter 2 for more information).

Postmarketing observational study: This is the process of monitoring and evaluating the safety of marketed health product using a variety of methods. Their purpose is generally to study large populations of users in ordinary practice with the aim of identifying adverse drug reactions that had been missed, before marketing because clinical trials were too small, too short, or did not always reflect real life (see Chapter 3 for more information).

Power, statistical power: This represents the probability that a statistical test will reject the null hypothesis when it is false in favor of a specified alternative hypothesis. Statistical power is the complementary probability of the Type II or b error. The statistical power defines, for example, the capability of a statistical test to reveal a given difference between two treatments, if this difference really exists. Power depends on the size of the difference we wish to detect, the chosen risk of Type I error, and the number of subjects included in the study.

Pragmatic trial: This type of trial consists in using pragmatic criteria chosen a priori, to assess the overall therapeutic value of a treatment compared to an already existing treatment. This kind of trial thus differs in its principle and objectives from an *explanatory clinical trial*, which seeks to demonstrate the intrinsic efficacy and/or tolerance of a treatment under standardized conditions. Ideally, a pragmatic trial is conducted after a Phase III trial, when the treatment and strategies to compare have already been in use for some time and is well-known by the medical practitioners. Treatments are allocated at random, as in an explanatory trial, but the nature of these treatments is known to both patients and health-care providers, which allows the normal therapeutic relationship to be taken into account. In this way, the prescriber can be guided in making his or her therapeutic decisions with full knowledge of the prescription context. The absence of blinding may, however, be a limitation if the assessment of the judgment criterion is subjective. In the strictest sense, this type of trial does not leave open the possibility of not reaching a conclusion. The treatment with the best results is adopted (balancing the advantages and disadvantages) without a statistical test or the possibility of nondecision (which corresponds, in the extreme, to accepting a Type II error of 0% and a Type I error of 100%). On the other hand, minimizing Type III error is an error that would consist of adopting the worse of the two options, requires calculation and recruitment of a sufficient number of subjects.

Prediction interval: This represents the set of possible values of a given parameter having a given prechosen probability of being observed in a sample of size *n*, assuming knowledge of the true value of this parameter. *Example: If the probability of occurrence of a pancytopenia over the course of a treatment is 1%, 10 cases can be expected if a sample of 1000 persons is followed.* The method of calculation is similar to that of a confidence interval except that the reasoning is reversed: a confidence interval is constructed around an observed parameter and is assumed to include (with a given probability) the true, unknown value of this parameter.

Prevalence: This is the number of cases of an event recorded in a population during a given period of time. The prevalence of a disease includes cases occurring during the study period (*incident cases*) and the cases occurring prior to this period that have yet not recovered. Prevalence measured in a population is thus always higher than incidence except when the duration of the disease is very short; in this case, the prevalence and the incidence tend to be identical. For the beginner, the term "prevalence" is often used to designate a prevalence rate (e.g., a prevalence of 8 per 1000).

Prevalence rate: This is the number of cases reported in a population during a given period, compared to the number of individuals at risk in the population. This rate includes cases appearing during the period of interest (incident cases) and the cases occurring prior to this period that have not yet recovered.

Preventability: This term is highly important in pharmacovigilance where it was observed that many adverse drug reactions could be preventable (see Foreword of this book). This term is referring to the avoidable character of particular adverse effects of a therapeutic strategy, usually a medicinal treatment. An adverse effect that would not have occurred had the therapeutic attitude conformed to the most commonly recognized recommendations (e.g., regarding whether or not to treat, the choice of treatment, dose, duration, etc.) is said to be "*avoidable*" or "*preventable*." A study of preventability seeks to identify, enumerate, and describe the adverse effects that can be prevented and to propose actions to ensure this prevention to diminish the risk associated with medicinal treatments.

Probability: This is the relative frequency defining the number of times an event is expected to occur or a hypothesis is expected to be verified over a large number of attempts, approaching infinity. A probability is generally expressed as a proportion between 0 and 1, often converted to a percentage from 0% to 100%.

Proper use: This represents the prescription or use of a health product conforming to the recommendations. The proper use concerns the prescriber (respecting the Canadian product monograph and medical references as to the indications, contraindications, dosage, length of treatment, and others), as well as the patient (respecting oral or written recommendations regarding both prescribed and nonprescribed health products).

Proportion: This represents the number of subjects presenting a given characteristic divided by the total number of subjects in the study population. A proportion can vary from 0 to 1, and can be converted into a percentage by multiplying it by 100% or into a rate by multiplying it by a power of 10. *For example, 16 cases observed during 1 year in a sample of 827 subjects is equivalent to a proportion of 16/827 = 0.0193* or *1.93% or an annual incidence rate of 19.3 per 1000.*

Prospective: This term concerns the future. This term is applied to studies in which a population is followed from a given date to detect events likely to occur after this date. A cohort study is thus prospective. The seemingly redundant term "*prospective cohort*" is sometimes used to designate a cohort whose subjects are identified and included after the beginning of the study and followed into the future. Such a cohort is thus the opposite of an "*historical cohort.*"

Prospective study: This consists in any epidemiological study in which the subjects are followed after their inclusion to study the possible appearance of a phenomenon. This term is thus synonymous with "cohort study" and can be based on the descriptive analysis of a single cohort or an etiologic analysis comparing two or more cohorts.

Protective effect: This represents a diminution of the risk of occurrence of an adverse event related to exposure to a factor or to the presence of a characteristic. In controlled studies with a reference group, a protective effect can be shown when a relative risk or odds ratio is significantly lower than 1.

Protocol: This document is describing the rationale, objectives, approach, and statistical methods of a trial and defines the conditions under which the trial will be carried out and analyzed. This definition also applies to epidemiological studies, including observational approaches. The existence of a protocol (which formalizes the procedure to make it reproducible by other observers) does not necessarily imply the introduction of constraints. This would be the case if the protocol imposed an additional element as a requirement for the study that would affect the normal conditions of care or the natural course of events.

Protopathic bias: This is the distortion of the estimate of the association between the exposure to a risk factor (e.g., the use of a specific health product) and the occurrence of an adverse event linked to the fact that the exposure actually started after the occurrence of the event, or at least after the first appearance of its manifestations. In the most pronounced and restrictive form of this bias, the use or prescription of the drug may even be motivated by the appearance of the first symptoms of the disease of interest. *Example: A cardiovascular drug could be wrongly accused of causing pulmonary fibrosis if it is frequently prescribed for dyspnea, which is, in fact, the first sign of pulmonary fibrosis.*

QALYs acronym for "Quality Adjusted Life Years": The expression of QALYs represents the balances in the number of years of life gained due to the implementation of a therapeutic strategy against the quality of the subject's life during the same period. In this way, a treatment ensuring a survival duration that is shorter but of better quality than another could be considered superior in a comparison expressed in QALYs. For many types of ailments, notably in cardiology and oncology, scores allow quantification of the discomfort felt by the patient, and thus a conversion of survival duration into number of QALYs. Expression in QALYs is particularly used in cost-utility studies.

Qualitative variable: They are variables that can take only discrete values that have no quantitative relationship to one another (e.g., sex, blood type, race, and others)? These are often permanent and characterize an individual.

Quantitative variable: Continuous variable or discrete variable.

Random: This is a situation in which an outcome is not systematically the result of an intervention (e.g., the prescription of a given health product) but is subject to chance and can be described by an appropriate probability model.

Examples: random selection of the controls for a study, random occurrence of an adverse event, and others.

Random error: This represents the deviation of the value of a parameter estimated in a sample from its true value. As opposed to bias, this deviation is not systematically in a given direction, but assumes a random character and may be described by an appropriate probability model. Therefore, the measurement of a parameter in a randomly chosen sample may assume a certain number of values compared to the true value that would be measured in the entire reference population. This set of possible values, reflecting the sampling variation, can be predicted by an appropriate probability distribution and constitutes the *prediction interval* for the measurement of this parameter. *Example: If the risk of thrombocytopenia associated with a medical treatment is 3 per 1000, six cases can be expected to occur in a follow-up of 2000 treated patients.* In the same way, the construction of a confidence interval around the value measured in a sample minimizes the risk of erroneous conclusion with respect to the true value of the parameter. For more information, the readers may wish to consult the ICH-E9 guideline on the statistical principle for clinical trial.

Randomization: This is a major concept in biostatistics and represents the decision or designation depending wholly on chance. In a clinical trial, for example, randomization is used to decide with a table of random numbers or a computerized procedure which of the compared treatments each subject will receive, without subjective intervention. Randomization is the only method that guarantees a balanced distribution among groups of known or unknown variables likely to bias the planned analysis. It is only within this framework that statistical tests are strictly reliable. For more information, the readers may wish to consult the ICH-E9 guideline on the statistical principle for clinical trial.

Rate: This consists in the quantification of the frequency of an event in a population per unit of time. The definition of a rate always includes a reference to time (e.g., an incidence rate of 6 cases per 10,000 subjects per year). When follow-up time is not the same for all subjects in the studied population, the number of cases of the event is often compared to a sum of person-times sometimes called *population time* (e.g., 5 cases per 1000 person-years). This denominator is obtained by summing the follow-up or exposure times of all of the subjects in the population. An important characteristic of a rate is the fact that the cases (e.g., the subjects having presented the event) forming the numerator come from the population represented by the denominator. In other words, only those subjects considered a priori susceptible to presenting the event and observed in a manner that guarantees identification of the event should be included in the denominator. For more information, the readers may wish to consult the ICH-E9 guideline on the statistical principle for clinical trial.

Ratio: This represents the division of one quantity by another. This very general term can, for example, express the relative size of two populations (e.g., ratio of elderly subjects/young subjects, sex ratio of males/females, benefit/risk ratio of a health product). Unlike a rate or proportion, a ratio can refer to two measurements carried out on different populations: incidence rate ratio (comparing two incidence rates), risk ratio (comparing two risks), odds ratio (comparing two odds), and others. In pharmacoepidemiology and pharmacovigilance the ratio of the most frequently used is the benefit/risk ratio. For the approval for marketing a new health product by a regulatory agency the benefits should outweigh the risk.

Rationale: Reasoning justifying the implementation of a study or the performance of an analysis.

Recall bias: This is an important term in pharmacoepidemiology study that is related to information bias in which subjects are likely to recall the event or exposure of interest with a different degree of accuracy according to the comparison group to which they belong. *Example: In a case-control study investigating the association between a given health product and a congenital malformation, mothers of malformed children (the cases) will tend, during an interview, to have a better recollection of health products taken at the beginning of their pregnancy than mothers of normal children (the controls). This can falsely increase the value of the odds ratio estimated in this study. Similarly, in a cohort study, subjects treated with a given health product could have better recollection of an adverse event than non-exposed subjects.* A selection bias only occurs when the recollection deviates systematically in a given direction. If the interviewed subject's memory is imprecise or poorly guided by the interviewer, but not in a systematic manner, the result is a random error that leads to a loss of precision but not a recall bias.

Rechallenge: This is a term used in imputability to designate the voluntary or involuntary resuming of a subject's treatment with a health product (under similar conditions of dose, duration, etc.) suspected of having previously caused an adverse event in this subject. Rechallenge is termed *positive* if the adverse event recurs, *negative* if it does not, and *inconclusive* if the conditions (e.g., dosage, associated treatments, disease evolution, etc.) are not the same for the repeat of the treatment. This term is also very important in the causality assessment of an adverse event. For more information, the readers may wish to consult the ICH-E2A; the electronic link is provided at the end of this book.

Record linkage: This is the process of assembling the information contained in two or more complementary files that are usually computerized, in such a way as to allow epidemiological analyses. For example, the data from a disease registry (see Chapter 2 for more information) can be used to select subjects having presented a given illness, and their possible prior exposure to a health product can be ascertained from prescription records.

Conversely, prescription records can be used to identify persons being or having been treated with a health product and hospital records can serve to identify persons hospitalized for a given event. The technique of record linkage attempts to complete the data available on each of the study subjects. It is therefore important that the records refer to the same reference population and that there is a way to clearly identify an individual in the various sets of records.

Reference population, reference group: This represents a group of subjects not exposed to the risk factor of interest and, ideally, similar to the exposed group in all other respects. The reference group is used to estimate a *reference risk* that will then be compared to the *absolute risk* measured in the exposed subjects. The ideal reference group is formed by random selection in the same source population from which the studied group arose. If this is not possible, which is generally the case in pharmacoepidemiology the comparability of the two groups must be verified with respect to the main variables capable of biasing the measurement and proposed comparison. For more information, the readers may wish to consult the ICH-E9 guideline on the statistical principle for clinical trial.

Reference risk: This represents the risk measured in a population, called the *reference population*, which resembles the exposed population in all respects except that its members have not been exposed to the factor under study. This is, for example, the risk measured in the control (comparison) group in a clinical trial or cohort study. The reference risk is a fundamental parameter in pharmacoepidemiology because it is the only one that quantifies the risk for a subject who has not been exposed to the health product of interest. The reference risk can be very different from the risk measured in the general population.

Registry, register: As already explained in Chapter 2, this system consists on regularly collecting and recording, in an organized manner, all cases of a given event (usually a disease) in a given geographical area (e.g., town, region, country, etc.). The creation of a registry presupposes the implementation of means to guarantee completeness of data collection. In pharmacoepidemiology, registries (e.g., of congenital malformations, cancer, or from those taking the same health product [drug registry]) are valuable sources of data to measure incidence rates or conduct a case-control study, for example. In pharmacovigilance a registry is often used for the active surveillance of an adverse drug reaction.

Regression analysis: This represents a statistical technique consisting of finding the mathematical model that most adequately predicts the value of a dependent variable y given the value(s) of one or more independent variable(s) $x1, x2, \ldots, xj$. The simplest model is the linear type, $y = bx$ or $y = a + bx$. The data analysis in epidemiology and pharmacoepidemiology often uses other models, such as the logistic or Cox models. For more information, the readers may wish to consult the ICH-E9 guideline on the statistical principle for clinical trial.

Regression coefficient: This is a coefficient that affects the value of an independent variable in a regression model to best predict the value of another, dependent variable. *For example, if the value of the dependent variable y is predicted by that of the independent variable x according to the equation:* $y = a + bx$, *b is the regression coefficient of the variable x.* For more information, the readers may wish to consult the ICH-E9 guideline on the statistical principle for clinical trial.

Relative risk: This is an important term in pharmacoepidemiology and is calculated by dividing the risk measured in an exposed population (the *absolute risk*) by that measured in a reference population similar in all respects except that its members were not exposed (the *reference risk*) (see text in Chapter 3). *Example: If the risk of aplastic anemia measured in a population treated by a drug (oncologic drug for example) is 12.6/100,000 and the reference risk in a nonexposed population for the same period is 7/1,000,000, the relative risk is* $(12.6/100{,}000)/(7/1{,}000{,}000) = 18$. *We speculate that the use of this health product during the period under consideration multiplies the risk of aplastic anemia by 18.* The relative risk measures the strength of the association between the exposure to a risk factor (e.g., a drug treatment) and the occurrence of an event. A value not significantly different from 1 indicates the absence of association, a value significantly greater than 1 indicates an increased risk linked to exposure, and a value significantly less than 1 indicates a protective effect due to exposure. The more the value of the relative risk differs from 1, the stronger the association. It is always preferable to give the corresponding one- or two-sided confidence interval with the value calculated for the relative risk. *Example: In the above example, the two-sided 95% confidence interval for the calculated value of 18 is (0.4; 31.2); this means that the true value of the relative risk associated with the exposure has 95 chances in 100 of being included within these two limits.* For more information, the readers may wish to consult the ICH-E9 guideline on the statistical principle for clinical trial.

Required sample size: This is the number of subjects that should be included in a controlled study (e.g., clinical trial, cohort, or case-control study), to guarantee at least a given probability (called *statistical power*) of rejecting the tested null hypothesis with a statistic test, if this hypothesis is proved to be false. The calculation of required sample size presupposes precise specification of the tested null hypothesis and alternative hypothesis, as well as the type of statistic test envisaged and the accepted level of Type I error. The choice of a one-sided comparison test generally results in a smaller sample size than a two-sided test. The calculation of required sample size is most often derived from statistical tests based on the normal distribution. For more information, the readers may wish to consult the ICH-E9 guideline on the statistical principle for clinical trial.

Retrospective: This is a kind of epidemiologic study that is interested by the past, or looking into the past. This term is the antonym of "*prospective*." The distinction between the two terms is based on the temporal directionality of the analysis and not on the period concerned (i.e., a prospective study can be based on prerecorded data). A prospective analysis begins with exposure to a risk factor and investigates the possible later occurrence of a given event. A retrospective analysis begins with the occurrence of an event and investigates the subject's possible prior exposure to a given risk factor. For more information, the readers may wish to consult the ICH-E9 guideline on the statistical principle for clinical trial.

Retrospective study: This is a kind of epidemiological study in which the possible cause or determinants of an event (a disease, symptom, and others) are investigated in the past history of subjects having presented this event (see text). This type of study may be controlled (a case-control study) or noncontrolled. It is therefore incorrect to consider "retrospective study" and "case-control study" as being synonymous terms, as some authors suggest. Similarly, it is incorrect to use the term "*retrospective study*" to designate any study based on prerecorded data. Retrospective denotes the temporal directionality of the analysis (beginning with the observed event and investigating possible previous exposure to a given risk factor) and not the fact that the event of interest has already occurred. For more information, the readers may wish to consult the ICH-E9 guideline on the statistical principle for clinical trial.

Reverse causality bias, cart versus horse bias: This type of bias consists of falsely concluding a causal relationship of the type A = B when the relationship, if it exists, is of type B = A. Reverse causality bias is to be feared when the data do not permit precise analysis of the chronology of events, such as in a cross-sectional study. For more information please consult Chapter 3.

Risk, hazard: This represents the probability that an event will occur at a time t when it has not occurred at time $t - 1$. In pharmacoepidemiology, this term designates the probability that a subject (whether exposed to a drug or not) will present an event at any given time, knowing that the subject had not presented it in the preceding time interval. The risk is often estimated from the incidence rate for the period of interest. *Example: If the annual incidence rate of an event measured in a population is 2.5 per 1000, the risk for a subject during a 2-month period will be (2.5/1000) × (2/12) = 0.00042 or 4.2/10,000.* Inferring an individual estimate (the risk) from a population estimate (the incidence rate) can lead to errors of interpretation if possible variations in the risk over time or among subjects are not taken into account. For more information, the readers may wish to consult the ICH-E9 guideline on the statistical principle for clinical trial.

Risk–benefit ratio: This is a very important concept related to the authorization for marketing of a new health product or a known health product for a new indication. This represents a consideration of therapeutic benefit when judging the acceptability of the risk associated with a medicinal or nonmedicinal treatment. The concept can be applied either at the level of the individual (i.e., the acceptability of the strategy for a given patient) or the population, by comparing, in a group of subjects, the expected or observed results in terms of therapeutic benefit and the risk of adverse effects.

Risk difference, excess risk, attributable risk: This consists in a difference between the risk measured in an exposed population (the *absolute risk*) and that measured in a nonexposed population (the *reference risk*). This difference quantifies the increase in risk associated with exposure. *Example: If the risk of thrombocytopenia measured in a cohort exposed to a given drug is 18/10,000, while the risk measured in a nonexposed cohort is 3/10,000, the risk difference for thrombocytopenia is 15/10,000.* For many authors, the terms "*excess risk*" and "*attributable risk*" should not be used synonymously with "*risk difference*" because the first two imply that the increase in risk observed in the exposed subjects can only have been induced by the exposure. Such a conclusion would be permissible within the context of an experimental study comparing two populations that are identical with respect to the factors that could influence the measurement; this is not necessarily the case in an observational study. For more information, the readers may wish to consult the ICH-E9 guideline on the statistical principle for clinical trial.

Risk factor: This important element in pharmacoepidemiology represents the characteristic associated with an increased probability of occurrence of an event or disease. This characteristic can be inherent to the individual (e.g., age, sex, genetic trait, and others), or linked to a disease, environmental factor, diet, drug use, family history, and others. The term "*risk factor*" does not imply the existence of a causal relationship between the presence of the factor and the occurrence of the event or disease. A risk factor can only be validly identified with a controlled study (i.e., if this factor is overrepresented among the subjects presenting the event compared with those not presenting it). Chapter 4 provides good concrete examples of this important term.

Risk ratio: This is the relationship between two risks, generally estimated in different populations. The ratio of the risk estimated in the exposed (*absolute risk*) to the risk measured in the nonexposed (*reference risk*) represents the particular case of the *relative risk*. For more information regarding this term, please review Chapter 3.

Sample: This represents a subgroup of a population selected for the purposes of a study. If the results of a measurement are to be extrapolated to a larger population, this subgroup should be as representative as possible of this population, at least with respect to the principal characteristics that can influence the parameter to be measured. Ideally, a sample should be formed by drawing subjects at random from the entire reference population. Because this is rarely feasible in pharmacoepidemiology, the possibility of selection bias should be kept in mind.

Sampling: It is an operation leading to the selection of a sample of subjects from a reference population.

The validity of statistical inference requires that sample subjects be representative of the population to which the results of the measurement(s) are to be extrapolated. From this point of view, there are three major sampling methods:

- *Random sampling*, which consists of sampling at random from the reference population. If the sample size is sufficiently large, the influence of sampling variation becomes negligible, which guarantees the representativeness of the study sample and eliminates the possibility of selection bias.
- *Systematic* (or *pseudo-random*) *sampling*, in which the selection of subjects is not random, but follows a system based on a criterion deemed to be independent of the studied phenomenon. *For example, it is possible to select one subject in five during a day of consultation of all neurological services of a given country.*
- *Nonrandom sampling*, in which the selection of subjects obeys neither a random nor a systematic process (e.g., selection of patients who agree to answer a questionnaire).
    - While this method is simpler to put into practice, it rarely ensures the representativeness of the sample and is therefore susceptible to selection bias.

Sampling fraction: This represents the ratio of the size of a sample (usually selected for a survey) to that of the population from which the sample was drawn, and to which the results of the measurement will generally be extrapolated. The sampling fraction is most often expressed as a percentage or a rate (*sampling rate*). *For example, a survey of the use of psychotropic medications consisted of interviewing 2040 adult subjects. On the basis of a total population of 4 million adults in the Province of Quebec, the sampling fraction is:* $(2040/4{,}000{,}000) \times 100\% = 0.05\%$. The sampling fraction is a fundamental parameter for judging the statistical stability of inferences made from surveys; notably, it is used in the calculation of a confidence interval around an estimate.

Seeding study: This is a pharmacoepidemiologic study being conducted for scientific purposes, when the principal (or even the only) objective for its sponsor is an increase in the number of prescriptions or the market share of the health product concerned. The term *seeding* applies principally to studies of health already on (or about to enter) the market, which therefore enter into the framework of Phase IV studies. In seeding or implantation studies, the recruitment, with honoraria, of a certain number of clinician-researchers is supposed to induce a somewhat-lasting habit of preferential prescription.

Except in a few obvious cases, it is not always easy to recognize whether a study has a promotional objective or whether it is a scientific study that may lead to increased market share through its positive outcomes.

Selection bias, sample distortion bias: This is a distortion of the estimate of the association between a risk factor (e.g., use of a drug) and the occurrence of an event, resulting from measurements made in a sample that is not representative of the population to which the results are to be extrapolated. A selection bias occurs when the event of interest is over or underrepresented in the sample as the result of a systematic error in selection. This is the case, for example, in a cohort study if the protocol leads to preferential selection of subjects (from the source population) that have a greater or lesser risk of presenting the event. In a case-control study, selection bias causes the subjects (cases or controls) to be nonrepresentative of the source population with respect to exposure to the factor of study.

Sensitivity: This represents a diagnostic test used to determine the proportion of *true positives* (i.e., diseased patients for whom the test is positive). This is calculated by dividing the number of *true positives* (a) by the number of times ($a + c$) the test has been administered to patients suffering from the disease:

	Diseased	Nondiseased
Positive test	a	b
Negative test	c	d
	$a + c$	$b + d$

A test whose sensitivity is 1 (100%) is positive every time the disease is present, that is, gives no *false negatives*. By analogy, the sensitivity of a method of detection of an adverse effect is the proportion of cases of the effect identified by this method in a population. *Example: If 15 cases of liver injury associated with a drug were spontaneously reported when 112 cases actually occurred, the sensitivity of the surveillance system is 15/112 or 0.13.*

Sensitivity testing, sensitivity analysis: This is a statistical method that uses a model to study the effect of changing the value(s) of one or more variable(s) on the final results. Such testing is frequently used in decision-making strategies, for example, when calculating the attributable number of cases or the number of subjects to include in a study, under different hypotheses of the value of the risk in the exposed persons.

Serious: According to the regulatory definition from the ICH and the Foods and Drug Regulations, serious is an adjective that usually applies to an event or adverse effect that is fatal, or life threatening, which causes hospitalization or prolongation of hospitalization, permanent or temporary functional disability or incapacity, cancer or congenital anomaly. This term thus appraises the consequences of the event or effect, whereas *severe* quantifies its intensity. Definition of *serious* can be found in ICH E2A proposing the following consequences of an event to be deemed serious:

- Death.
- Threat to the patient's life at the moment of occurrence of the event.
- Necessity for hospital admission or prolongation of hospitalization.
- Significant and lasting disability (meaning the impossibility of carrying out normal tasks of daily living).
- Congenital abnormality or perinatal crisis.
- Obvious risk to the patient, requiring treatment or intervention to prevent any of the five complications noted above.

Severity: This represents the intensity of an adverse event, unlike the *seriousness*, presupposes its consequences in terms of mortality or morbidity. This defines an adverse event or symptom as being:

- *Mild* if it does not affect the daily activity of the patient.
- *Moderate* if this activity is disturbed.
- *Severe* if this activity is made impossible.

Side effect: This consists in an unwanted manifestation related to a pharmacological property of a health product. This may be a particular expression of its main pharmacological effect (used therapeutically) or a subsidiary property. A side effect may or may not have harmful consequences.

Signal: This represents an event exceeding a predetermined frequency or intensity level, recognized as worthy of attention during surveillance (see Chapter 4 for a concrete example of signal detection to ease the understanding of this term). In practice, this term is used when the value of a parameter (e.g., number of cases of an event, incidence rate, and others) differs from expected or normal values. After validation (e.g., *signal strengthening*), a signal is an *alert* that should lead to decision-making or the implementation of an appropriate study. In pharmacovigilance, "*signal*" designates reported information on a possible causal relationship between an adverse event and a health product, the relationship being unknown or incompletely documented previously. Usually more than a single report is required to generate a signal, depending on the seriousness of the event and the quality of the information provided in these reports in terms of medical history, labs, concomitant medication, and others.

Simplified clinical trial (SCT): This is a specific kind of experimental design that conserves the random allocation of compared treatments, but having less rigorous criteria for subject selection, surveillance procedures, and control of recorded data to simplify the implementation of the trial, reduce its cost, eventually include a greater number of subjects, and approximate the usual conditions of care. *Simplified clinical trials* cannot replace the clinical trials required to obtain NDA and are generally undertaken after this has been obtained. Certain types of simplified trials are similar to a *pragmatic trial*. In all cases, they are prospective studies based on the observation of one or more cohort(s).

Source population: This is a very important concept in pharmacoepidemiology and represents the population from which the study subjects are selected. The source population can be defined by geographical area (e.g., city, region, country, and others), in which case it corresponds to the general population, or by a sociodemographic characteristic (e.g., the presence of a disease, the fact of treatment with a given drug, and others). When the results of an estimate made in a group of study subjects are extrapolated to the entire population, the source population correspond to the target population.

Specific rate: This represents the incidence or prevalence rate calculated in a given subgroup of a population. In *stratification* and *standardization* methods, for example, the specific rate is calculated for each of the subgroups defined according to the value of a given variable, or the presence or absence of a given criterion.

Specificity: For a diagnostic test, this represents the proportion of *true negatives* (i.e., nondiseased patients for whom the test is negative). This is calculated by dividing the number of *true negatives* (d) by the number of times ($b + d$) that the test has been administered to subjects not suffering from the disease (see table below).

	Diseased	**Nondiseased**
Positive test	a	b
Negative test	c	d
	$a + c$	$b + d$

A test whose specificity is 1 (100%) is always negative when the disease is absent, that is, gives no *false positives*. By analogy, the specificity of a surveillance method is its capacity to detect only the events corresponding to the case definition, without false positives.

Sponsor: This word represents the individual or organization supporting a research project (study or trial) and interested in its results.

Stratification: This approach consists in dividing a sample or population into several subgroups according to the distribution of a given criterion (e.g., age, socioeconomic status, number of associated health products, and others). The calculation of *specific rates* for each of these subgroups, defined according to the presence of a factor or the value of a variable, can be used to assess the influence of this factor or the value of this variable on the measurement. *Example: Stratification according to age can reveal the fact that an excess mortality measured in a treated population is actually due to an overrepresentation of older subjects in this population (if a comparison with* *the equivalent age groups in a reference population does not show a significant difference*). Stratification also makes it possible to detect the possible modifying effect of a given variable.

Surrogate endpoint: This endpoint is very important in clinical research and is often difficult to select and needs judgment in the selection of criterion that predicts the evolution of another more robust criterion, and used as a substitute when the latter proves difficult or inconvenient, notably for reasons of sample size, duration of study, or ethics. This may be a biological criterion (e.g., blood glucose level, blood cells count), a test (e.g., blood arterial pressure, electromyography), an imaging method (e.g., X-ray, scan or MRI results, visualization of a tumor), etc. *For example, hormone-replacement therapy in menopausal women seeks to reduce the risk of fracture in this population, notably due to osteoporosis. To judge the efficacy of a new treatment using the robust criterion of a lessening of the risk of compression fractures would require a follow-up of more than 10 years. It is permissible, at least at the beginning, to judge this efficacy by the comparative evolution of the bone mineral density, which allows for a considerably shorter study.* A surrogate endpoint is only acceptable if:

- Its evaluation is reliable, unambiguous, and reproducible.
- There is a clear and well-established relationship between the surrogate endpoint and the relevant clinical criterion.
- It has been demonstrated that its evolution is correlated, in a reciprocal manner, with that of the relevant clinical criterion (strong predictive value); this implies that a favorable or unfavorable evolution of the surrogate endpoint predicts an evolution in the same direction (and if possible of the same amplitude) of the relevant clinical criterion, and this correlation has been demonstrated in the population under study (see ICH E3 for more information). Surrogate endpoints are also used in pharmacovigilance studies (e.g., electromyogram for peripheral neuropathy, specific activity of transaminases for hepatitis, etc.).

Survey: This represents the selection of a given number of individuals from a population (the reference population) to study their characteristics, state of health or well-being, behavior or opinion about a given health problem. Surveying is an inferential procedure in that the measurements taken from a sample are usually extrapolated to the entire reference population from which the subjects were gathered. This requires that the study sample is representative of the reference population regarding the main variables likely to bias the measurement or analysis. There are numerous methods for achieving representativeness: random selection of subjects from the entire reference population (simple *random sampling*), selection of a certain number of group of individuals (families or collective groups) from the population (*cluster sampling*), or surveying in subgroups chosen from the population according to a given parameter such as age (*stratified sampling*). In all cases, the relation of the sample size to the reference population (*survey fraction* or *rate*) determines the precision of the estimate and the validity of the inference.

Survival bias: This consists in the bias in which the fact of being exposed to the factor of interest modifies the duration of survival and thus a subject's probability of being included in a study. As a result, exposure can be over- or underrepresented among survivors, which risks biasing estimation. *Example: If a drug causes cardiac arrhythmia with an immediately fatal outcome, the exposed cases (treated with this drug) will have a lower probability of living long enough to be interviewed than those who were not exposed. This will likely result in the underestimation of exposure among cases and thus the risk associated with this health product. The consequences would be the reverse if the cardiac arrhythmia induced by this health product had a lower early mortality than that induced by other causes.* For more information about bias, please consult Chapter 3; furthermore there are concrete examples of bias and their impact in the interpretation of results in Chapter 4.

Synergism, synergy: This represents the type of interaction in which the effect of one factor on the studied variable is increased by the presence of another factor. In pharmacology, we generally make the following distinctions:

- *Additive effect*, in which the resulting effect is equal to the sum of the effects of each of the health products considered separately (also called additive effect).
- *Partial additive effect*, in which the resulting effect is greater than the effect of the health product considered in isolation, but less than the sum of the effects of each of the health products administered.
- *Synergism*, in which the resulting effect is greater than the algebraic sum of the effects of each the health products considered in isolation.
- In the strictest sense, "*additive effect*" refers to two health products acting by the same mechanism, whereas for *synergism* they act at different sites. In epidemiology, "*synergism*" or "*synergy*" usually indicates a multiplicative model in which the resulting effect is greater than the sum of the effects of each of the factors considered separately.

Target population: This term has two different meanings and is used to designate:

- A population addressed by a public health intervention, particularly one that is likely to receive a given treatment. This target population does not necessarily correspond to the population actually treated, called the *joint population.*
- The population to which the results of a study or estimates made in a sample can be legitimately extrapolated.

Therapeutic benefit: This consists in the expected or measured improvement in the state of health or well-being of a subject or population, related to the implementation of a therapeutic strategy, whether or not this involves a medical treatment. This improvement can be immediate or delayed, transient or permanent, but must be relevant in terms of individual benefit or public health and assessed according to sufficiently robust criteria (e.g., decreased mortality or morbidity, improved quality of life, etc.).

Therapeutic drug monitoring: This represents the use of plasma drug concentrations to adjust the dosage of a health product in individual patients, based on a range of target values, or on mathematical models derived from individual patients' pharmacokinetic parameters, or from population pharmacokinetic studies.

Therapeutic effect: This represents the measurable improvement in the state of health or well-being of a subject associated with the use of a health product and apparently explainable by one or more of its pharmacological properties. This improvement can be immediate or delayed, transient or permanent depending on the pharmacological properties of health product and the response to treatment by the patient.

Therapeutic index: This is particularly important for health products known to have a low therapeutic index, and this represents the ratio of the dose of a health product considered toxic to the dose considered therapeutically efficacious for a given indication. Theoretically, the greater the ratio, the easier the health product is to use. For health products with a low therapeutic index, the toxic dose is very close to the dose shown to be efficacious in a majority of subjects; the dosage should therefore be adjusted with great precision.

Time-window: This represents the interval of time considered relevant in the design or analysis of an epidemiological study (see case report in Chapter 4 for more information). In case-control studies, it is essential to define a priori the period during which possible exposure to the risk factor of interest will be investigated in the previous history of both cases and controls. *Example: If it is thought that liver injury cannot occur before the end of the first week nor after 2 months of continuous drug treatment, the only subjects considered to be exposed to the drug will be those whose treatment began after than 7 days but less than 61 days before the occurrence of the first symptoms of liver injury.* The time-window used to characterize an exposure is always defined with respect to an *index* or *reference date*, which can be, for example, the date of occurrence of the event or the first symptoms for the cases. An equivalent date must be defined for the controls. Similarly, in a cohort study, the time-window defines the period after the beginning of the exposure during which the occurrence of the event of interest will be investigated. *Example: An X-ray contrast media product is suspected of inducing hepatocarcinoma. Based on data available in the literature, this event may occur between 5 and 15 years after the injection of the health product. This interval forms an adequate time-window for comparing the incidence of this cancer in exposed and nonexposed populations.* The a priori choice of a time-window is difficult if the pathogenetic mechanism or the hazard function of the event of interest is poorly documented. This is particularly relevant since an inappropriate time-window can strongly bias the estimate of risk.

Toxic effect, toxic reaction: This consists in a harmful manifestation resulting from the administration of a toxic, supratherapeutic dose of a health product. This effect can be the result of a large dose over a short or extremely short period of time (*intoxication* or *acute toxicity*) or repeated doses resulting in an excessive cumulative dose (*cumulative* or *chronic toxicity*). The term more generally applies to manifestations resulting from too great a concentration of an active ingredient or one of its metabolites in a target tissue or organ. The therapeutic safety window of a given drug depends on the relationship between toxic and efficacious doses; this ratio is sometimes termed a "*therapeutic index*."

Traceability: This is very important for the follow-up of adverse drug reactions especially in the case of biosimilars and represents the capability of following the history of a package or a batch of a health product from its manufacture until its storage, dispensation, or administration to a subject. Ensuring the traceability of a product requires implementation of means by which all packages and their present or past users can be found at any time. Traceability has become a legal requirement for blood products and health product derived from human blood.

Treated: This term applied to a subject using a health product under conditions (e.g., of indication, dosage, duration of treatment, etc.), which allow the expectation of a therapeutic benefit. These conditions do not necessarily correspond to those characterizing the exposure, which place the subject at risk of presenting a given adverse effect. A patient can thus either be treated and exposed, treated and not exposed, or exposed and not treated (if the dose and/or duration of the treatment are not sufficient to expect a therapeutic benefit).

True negative: This represents subjects free from a disease that a test is supposed to detect, and for whom this test is negative (*see also*: negative predictive value, specificity).

True positive: This consists in subjects with a disease that a test is supposed to detect, and for whom this test is positive (see also: positive predictive value or sensitivity).

Two-sided test, two-tailed test: This is a statistical test in which the rejection area of the null hypothesis lies on either side of this hypothesis. The choice of a two-sided test is conservative in the sense that it requires inclusion of more subjects than a one-sided test, to have a given probability (*statistical power*) of detecting a given difference between the variables being compared. This test is nevertheless preferable whenever we are interested in exploring both sides of the rejection zone.

Type I error, alpha error: This represents the probability of wrongly rejecting the null hypothesis in favor of a prestated alternative hypothesis. When comparing two therapeutic strategies, for example, Type I error is the maximum risk we will accept of falsely finding a difference that does not in fact exist. The complement of the Type I error ($1 - \alpha$) represents the *confidence level* of the chosen conclusion.

Type II error, beta error: It is the probability of not rejecting the null hypothesis, although it is false in favor of a prestated alternative hypothesis. This is, for example, the risk of not detecting a given difference that in fact exists. The complement of this probability ($1 - \beta$) represents the power of the statistical test or study.

Type III error, gamma risk: This consists in a comparison of two values or treatments using a two-sided statistical test, the risk of concluding that one of them is superior to the other, when it is in fact inferior. Type III error is often associated with *pragmatic trials* (*see above*).

Underreporting, underreporting coefficient: This is often a problem in the analysis of spontaneous reporting and is the failure to report to a passive surveillance system a proportion of the cases of an adverse effect that have occurred during a given period in a given area. This may be caused by numerous factors: absence of motivation or time on the part of the observer, absence of diagnosis of the event, or nonattribution of the event to a health product. The effectiveness of spontaneous reporting can be quantified by the proportion of reported cases (the number of cases of adverse effects reported divided by the total number of cases occurring in the population during the same period). This proportion is by definition equal to 1 (100%) at the most and can be extremely low in certain cases, for example, when the adverse effect is well known and not serious. The inverse of this proportion is the *underreporting coefficient*, the factor by which the number of reported cases should be multiplied to estimate the number of cases that have actually occurred. *Example: 20 cases of arrythmia were reported in the second year of the availability of a health product on the market. It is later revealed that 100 cases actually occurred during this period. The proportion of reported cases is 20/100 = 0.20 (20%) and the underreporting coefficient is 100/20 = 5.* Unfortunately, although these concepts are useful in theoretical calculations and modeling, in practice it is rare to know the precise number of cases actually occurring, to be able to calculate the proportion of reported cases or the underreporting coefficient. It is only possible to make estimates of varying validity.

Unexpected adverse drug reaction, unexpected adverse effect: This is an important concept in pharmacoepidemiology and represents a harmful and undesirable manifestation attributed to a health product but not apparently connected with one of its known pharmacological properties of this health product. It is generally acknowledged that an unexpected adverse effect reveals one or more risk factor(s) inherent to certain patients (e.g., prior allergic sensitivity, metabolic anomaly, deficit of a given amino acid, a specific receptor population, etc.). The incidence of the effect can be low or very low, according to the distribution of these factors in the exposed population. The prior ignorance of these risk factors justifies the use of the term "*unexpected*" even if the mechanism can subsequently be established. An unexpected adverse effect is sometimes called a "Type B reaction." By extension and somewhat abusively, current international definitions tend to denote an *unlabeled effect* as "unexpected," that is, an effect not clearly mentioned in the most recent version of the product monograph, for example or in the investigator's brochure in a clinical trial.

Variable: This is an important concept in pharmacoepidemiology and represents the object of a measurement, which may take any value within previously defined limits (*continuous variable*) or several states according to the individuals or circumstances (*qualitative variable*). If the value of a variable is not modified by the presence of a factor or the value taken by another variable, we speak of an *independent variable*; in the contrary situation, the variable is said to be *dependent*.

Volunteer: This represents subjects willingly participating in clinical research after having freely consented, with full knowledge of the goals, constraints, and possible risks inherent in this research. It should be emphasized that a person cannot legally be made to participate in research without this consent having first been obtained. The subjects must sign a document named informed consent form (ICF) before enrolling in a clinical research.

Washout period: This period represents the complete elimination of the active principle of a drug at the conclusion of a period without treatment. A sufficiently long washout period is indispensable for bringing the study subjects back to their baseline status, that is, to assume that the active principle is no longer able to interfere with the proposed measurement. Such free intervals can be planned before inclusion of previously treated subjects, or, in the case of *crossover studies*, in between treatment sequences being compared.

REFERENCES

Begaud B. *Dictionary of Pharmacoepidemiology.* John Wiley & Sons Ltd; 2000.

CIOMS Working Group Pharmacovigilance (2016). Available at: https://cioms.ch/pharmacovigilance/becoming-the-cioms-member/.

Guideline for Good Clinical Practice E6 (R1); 1996. Available at: http://www.ich.org/fileadmin/Public_Web_Site/ICH_Products/Guidelines/Efficacy/E6_R1/Step4/E6_R1__Guideline.pdf.

Health Canada: Good Pharmacovigilance Practices (GVP) Guidelines (GUI-0102) (2013). Available at: https://www.canada.ca/content/dam/hc-sc/migration/hc-sc/dhp-mps/alt_formats/pdf/compli-conform/gmp-bpf/docs/gui-0102_gvp-eng.pdf.

ICH guideline E2B (R3) on electronic transmission of individual case safety reports (ICSRs) - data elements and message specification - implementation guide (2013). Available at: http://www.ema.europa.eu/docs/en_GB/document_library/Scientific_guideline/2009/09/WC500002767.pdf.

ICH Harmonized Tripartite Guideline. Clinical Safety Data Management: Definitions and Standards for Expedited Reporting E2A; 1994. Disponible à http://www.ich.org/fileadmin/Public_Web_Site/ICH_Products/Guidelines/Efficacy/E2A/Step4/E2A_Guideline.pdf.

ICH Harmonized Tripartite Guideline. Choice of Control Group and Related Issues in Clinical Trials (E10); 2000. Available at: www.ich.org//choice-ofcontrol-group-and-related-issues-in-clinical-trials.pdf.

ICH Topic E 3: Structure and Content of Clinical Study Reports (1996). Available at: http://www.ema.europa.eu/docs/en_GB/document_library/Scientific_guideline/2009/09/WC500002832.pdf.

Samet JM, Wipfli H, Platz EA, Bavspar N. A Dictionary of Epidemiology. In: Porta Miquel, ed. *American Journal of Epidemiology*. Fifth Edition 170. 2009:1449.

World Health Organization. Available at: http://www.who.int/topics/epidemiology/en/.

Annex 3

Food and Drug Act and Regulations*

A). Food and Drug Act.

Article 12:

No person shall sell any drug described in Schedule C or D unless the Minister has, in prescribed form and manner, indicated that the premises in which the drug was manufactured and the process and conditions of manufacture therein are suitable to ensure that the drug will not be unsafe for use. For more information on the Food and Drug Act, please consult the following link: http://laws-lois.justice.gc.ca/eng/acts/f-27/.

B). Regulations on Food and Drug: Part C-Drug: Division 1:

1) **Interdiction.**
   C.01.016 No manufacturer shall sell a drug unless the manufacturer complies with the conditions set out in Sections C.01.017 to C.01.019. For more information please consult the following link: http://laws-lois.justice.gc.ca/eng/regulations/C.R.C.%2C_c._870/.

2) **Serious Adverse Drug Reaction Reporting**
   C.01.017 The manufacturer shall submit to the Minister a report of all information relating to the following serious adverse drug reactions within 15 days after receiving or becoming aware of the information, whichever occurs first:
   (a) any serious adverse drug reaction that has occurred in Canada with respect to the drug; and
   (b) any serious unexpected adverse drug reaction that has occurred outside Canada with respect to the drug.

---

* Many of the articles have been truncated to retain and only the most relevant information. Please also note that only the most pertinent articles and regulations have been presented. For more information please consult the links from the Food and Drug Acts and Regulations included in the text.

3) Annual Summary Report and Case Reports
C.01.018

(a) The manufacturer shall prepare an annual summary report of all information relating to adverse drug reactions and serious adverse drug reactions to the drug that it received or became aware of during the previous 12 months.
(b) The annual summary report shall contain a concise, critical analysis of the adverse drug reactions and serious adverse drug reactions to the drug.
(c) In preparing the annual summary report, the manufacturer shall determine, on the basis of the analysis referred to in subsection (2), whether there has been a significant change in what is known about the risks and benefits of the drug during the period covered by the report and shall include its conclusions in this regard in the summary report.
(d) If, in preparing the annual summary report, the manufacturer concludes that there has been a significant change, it shall notify the Minister without delay, in writing, unless this has already been done.
(e) The Minister may, for the purposes of assessing the safety and effectiveness of the drug, request in writing for the manufacturer to submit to the Minister one or both of the following:
  (1) the annual summary reports;
  (2) the case reports relating to the adverse drug reactions and serious adverse drug reactions to the drugs that are known to the manufacturer.
(f) The Minister shall, after giving the manufacturer an opportunity to be heard, specify a period for the submission of the annual summary reports or case reports, or both, which are reasonable in the circumstances, and the manufacturer shall submit the reports within that period.

4) Issue-Related Summary Report
C.01.019

(a) The Minister may, for the purposes of assessing the safety and effectiveness of the drug, request in writing for the manufacturer to submit to the Minister an issue-related summary report.
(b) The report shall contain a concise, critical analysis of the adverse drug reactions and serious adverse drug reactions to the drug, as well as case reports of all or specified adverse drug reactions and serious adverse drug reactions to the drugs that are known to the manufacturer in respect of the issue that the Minister directs the manufacturer to analyze in the report.

(c) The Minister shall, after giving the manufacturer an opportunity to be heard, specify a period for the submission of the report that is reasonable in the circumstances. The Minister may only specify a period that is less than 30 days if the Minister needs the information in the report to determine whether the drug poses a serious and imminent risk to human health.

(d) The manufacturer shall submit the report within the specified period.

C). Division 5: Drugs for Clinical Trials Involving Human Subjects

1) Application for Authorization

C.05.005 An application by a sponsor for authorization to sell or import a drug for the purposes of a clinical trial under this Division shall be submitted to the Minister, signed and dated by the sponsor's senior medical or scientific officer in Canada and senior executive officer and shall contain the following information and documents:

(a) a copy of the protocol for the clinical trial;

(b) a copy of the statement, as it will be set out in each informed consent form, which states the risks and anticipated benefits arising to the health of clinical trial subjects as a result of their participation in the clinical trial;

(c) a clinical trial attestation, signed and dated by the sponsor's senior medical or scientific officer in Canada and senior executive officer, containing

- **(1)** the title of the protocol and the clinical trial number,
- **(2)** the brand name, the chemical name, or the code for the drug,
- **(3)** the therapeutic and pharmacological classifications of the drug,
- **(4)** the medicinal ingredients of the drug,
- **(5)** the nonmedicinal ingredients of the drug,
- **(6)** the dosage form of the drug,
- **(7)** the name, address, and telephone number and, if applicable, the facsimile number and electronic mail address of the sponsor,
- **(8)** if the drug is to be imported, the name, address and telephone number and, if applicable, the facsimile number, and electronic mail address of the sponsor's representative in Canada who is responsible for the sale of the drug,
- **(9)** for each clinical trial site, the name, address, and telephone number and, if applicable, the facsimile number and electronic mail address of the qualified investigator, if known at the time of submitting the application,

(10) for each clinical trial site, the name, address and telephone number and, if applicable, the facsimile number and electronic mail address of the research ethics board that approved the protocol referred to in paragraph (a) and approved an informed consent form containing the statement referred to in paragraph (b), if known at the time of submitting the application, and

(11) a statement

(A) that the clinical trial will be conducted in accordance with good clinical practices and these Regulations, and

(B) that all information contained in, or referenced by, the application is complete and accurate and is not false or misleading;For the complete information about this rule please consult the following link: http://laws-lois.justice.gc.ca/eng/regulations/C.R.C.%2C_c._870/.

2) Authorization
C.05.006

(a) Subject to subsection (c), a sponsor may sell or import a drug, other than a drug described in subsection (b), for the purposes of a clinical trial if

(1) the sponsor has submitted to the Minister an application in accordance with Section C.05.005;

(2) the Minister does not, within 30 days after the date of receipt of the application, send to the sponsor a notice in respect of the drug indicating that the sponsor may not sell or import the drug for any of the following reasons:

(A) that the information and documents in respect of the application

(i) were not provided in accordance with these Regulations, or

(ii) are insufficient to enable the Minister to assess the safety and risks of the drug or the clinical trial;

(B) that based on an assessment of the application, an assessment of any information submitted under Section C.05.009 or a review of any other information, the Minister has reasonable grounds to believe that

(i) the use of the drug for the purposes of the clinical trial endangers the health of a clinical trial subject or other person,

(ii) the clinical trial is contrary to the best interests of a clinical trial subject, or

(iii) the objectives of the clinical trial will not be achieved;

(3) for each clinical trial site, the sponsor has obtained the approval of the research ethics board in respect of the protocol referred to in paragraph C.05.005(a) and in respect of an informed consent form that contains the statement referred to in paragraph C.05.005(b); and

(4) before the sale or importation of the drug at a clinical trial site, the sponsor submits to the Minister the information referred to in subparagraphs C.05.005(c) (9) and (10) and paragraphs C.05.005(d) and (h), if it was not submitted in respect of that clinical trial site at the time of submitting the application.

(b) Subject to subsection (3), a sponsor may sell or import a drug for the purposes of a clinical trial in respect of

(1) a new drug that has been issued a notice of compliance under subsection C.08.004(a), if the clinical trial is in respect of a purpose or condition of use for which the notice of compliance was issued; or

(2) a drug, other than a new drug, which has been assigned a drug identification number under subsection C.01.014.2(1), if the clinical trial is in respect of a use or purpose for which the drug identification number was assigned.

(c) A sponsor may not sell or import a drug for the purposes of a clinical trial

(1) during the period of any suspension made under Section C.05.016 or C.05.017; or

(2) after a cancellation made under Section C.05.016 or C.05.017.

3) Sponsor's Obligations: Good Clinical Practices.

C.05.010 Every sponsor shall ensure that a clinical trial is conducted in accordance with good clinical practices and, without limiting the generality of the foregoing, shall ensure that

(a) the clinical trial is scientifically sound and clearly described in a protocol;

(b) the clinical trial is conducted, and the drug is used, in accordance with the protocol and this Division;

(c) systems and procedures that assure the quality of every aspect of the clinical trial are implemented;

(d) for each clinical trial site, the approval of a research ethics board is obtained before the clinical trial begins at the site;

(e) at each clinical trial site, there is no more than one qualified investigator;

(f) at each clinical trial site, medical care and medical decisions, in respect of the clinical trial, are under the supervision of the qualified investigator;

(g) each individual involved in the conduct of the clinical trial is qualified by education, training, and experience to perform his or her respective tasks;

(h) written informed consent, given in accordance with the applicable laws governing consent, is obtained from every person before that person participates in the clinical trial but only after that person has been informed of

  (1) the risks and anticipated benefits to his or her health arising from participation in the clinical trial, and

  (2) all other aspects of the clinical trial that are necessary for that person to make the decision to participate in the clinical trial;

(i) the requirements respecting information and records set out in Section C.05.012 are met; and

(j) the drug is manufactured, handled, and stored in accordance with the applicable good manufacturing practices referred to in Divisions 2–4 except Sections C.02.019, C.02.025, and C.02.026.

4) Serious Unexpected Adverse Drug Reaction Reporting
C.05.014

(a) During the course of a clinical trial, the sponsor shall inform the Minister of any serious unexpected adverse drug reaction in respect of the drug that has occurred inside or outside Canada as follows:

  (1) if it is neither fatal nor life threatening, within 15 days after becoming aware of the information; and

  (2) if it is fatal or life threatening, within 7 days after becoming aware of the information.

(b) The sponsor shall, within 8 days after having informed the Minister under paragraph (a) (2), submit to the Minister a complete report in respect of that information that includes an assessment of the importance and implication of any findings made.

(c) Sections C.01.016 to C.01.020 do not apply to drugs used for the purposes of a clinical trial.

5) Suspension and Cancellation
C.05.016

(a) Subject to subsection (b), the Minister shall suspend the authorization to sell or import a drug for the purposes of a clinical trial, in its entirety or at a clinical trial site, if the Minister has reasonable grounds to believe that

  (1) the sponsor has contravened these Regulations or any provisions of the Act relating to the drug;

  (2) any information submitted in respect of the drug or clinical trial is false or misleading;

  (3) the sponsor has failed to comply with good clinical practices; or

(4) the sponsor has failed to provide
(A) information or samples of the drug as required under Section C.05.009 or C.05.013, or
(B) information or a report under Section C.05.014.

(b) Subject to Section C.05.017, the Minister shall not suspend an authorization referred to in subsection (a) unless
(1) the Minister has sent to the sponsor a written notice of the intention to suspend the authorization that indicates whether the authorization is to be suspended in its entirety or at a clinical trial site and the reason for the intended suspension;
(2) the sponsor has not, within 30 days after receipt of the notice referred to in paragraph (a), provided the Minister with information or documents that demonstrate that the authorization should not be suspended on the grounds that
(A) the situation giving rise to the intended suspension did not exist, or
(B) the situation giving rise to the intended suspension has been corrected; and
(3) the Minister has provided the sponsor with the opportunity to be heard in paragraph (b).

(c) The Minister shall suspend the authorization by sending to the sponsor a written notice of suspension of the authorization that indicates the effective date of the suspension, whether the authorization is suspended in its entirety or at a clinical trial site and the reason for the suspension.

(d) If the Minister has suspended an authorization under subsection (1), the Minister shall
(1) reinstate the authorization in its entirety or at a clinical trial site, as the case may be, if within 30 days after the effective date of the suspension the sponsor provides the Minister with information or documents that demonstrate that the situation giving rise to the suspension has been corrected; or
(2) cancel the authorization in its entirety or at a clinical trial site, as the case may be, if within 30 days after the effective date of the suspension the sponsor has not provided the Minister with the information or documents referred to in paragraph (a).

D). Division 8: New Drugs

1) Definition:

C.08.001 For the purposes of the Act and this Division, *new drug* means
(a) a drug that contains or consists of a substance, whether as an active or inactive ingredient, carrier, coating, excipient, menstruum, or other component, which has not been sold as a drug in Canada for

sufficient time and in sufficient quantity to establish in Canada the safety and effectiveness of that substance for use as a drug;

(b) a drug that is a combination of two or more drugs, with or without other ingredients, and that has not been sold in that combination or in the proportion in which those drugs are combined in that drug, for sufficient time and in sufficient quantity to establish in Canada the safety and effectiveness of that combination and proportion for use as a drug; or

(c) a drug, with respect to which the manufacturer prescribes, recommends, proposes, or claims a use as a drug, or a condition of use as a drug, including dosage, route of administration, or duration of action and that has not been sold for that use or condition of use in Canada, for sufficient time and in sufficient quantity to establish in Canada the safety and effectiveness of that use or condition of use of that drug.

C.08.001.1 For the purposes of this Division.

Canadian reference product means

(a) a drug in respect of which a notice of compliance is issued under Section C.08.004 or C.08.004.01 and which is marketed in Canada by the innovator of the drug,

(b) a drug, acceptable to the Minister, which can be used for the purpose of demonstrating bioequivalence on the basis of pharmaceutical and, where applicable, bioavailability characteristics, where a drug in respect of which a notice of compliance has been issued under Section C.08.004 or C.08.004.01 cannot be used for that purpose because it is no longer marketed in Canada, or

(c) a drug, acceptable to the Minister, which can be used for the purpose of demonstrating bioequivalence on the basis of pharmaceutical and, where applicable, bioavailability characteristics, in comparison to a drug referred to in paragraph (a); (*produit de référence canadien*)For the complete information about this rule please consult the following link: http://laws-lois.justice.gc.ca/eng/regulations/C.R.C.%2C_c._870/.

2) Interdiction:

C.08.002

(a) No person shall sell or advertise a new drug unless

(1) the manufacturer of the new drug has filed with the Minister a new drug submission, an extraordinary use new drug submission, an abbreviated new drug submission, or an abbreviated extraordinary use new drug submission relating to the new drug that is satisfactory to the Minister;

(2) the Minister has issued, under Section C.08.004 or C.08.004.01, a notice of compliance to the manufacturer of the new drug in respect of the submission; and
(3) the notice of compliance in respect of the submission has not been suspended under Section C.08.006.

(b) A new drug submission shall contain sufficient information and material to enable the Minister to assess the safety and effectiveness of the new drug.
For the complete information about this rule please consult the following link: http://laws-lois.justice.gc.ca/eng/regulations/C.R.C.%2C_c._870/.

3) **Authorization:**
C.08.004

(a) Subject to Section C.08.004.1, the Minister shall, after completing an examination of a new drug submission or abbreviated new drug submission or a supplement to either submissions,
(1) if that submission or supplement complies with Section C.08.002, C.08.002.1, or C.08.003, as the case may be, and Section C.08.005.1, issue a notice of compliance, or
(2) if that submission or supplement does not comply with Section C.08.002, C.08.002.1, or C.08.003, as the case may be, or Section C.08.005.1, notify the manufacturer that the submission or supplement does not so comply.

(b) Where a new drug submission or abbreviated new drug submission or a supplement to either submissions does not comply with Section C.08.002, C.08.002.1, or C.08.003, as the case may be, or Section C.08.005.1, the manufacturer who filed the submission or supplement may amend the submission or supplement by filing additional information or material.For the complete information about this rule please consult the following link: http://laws-lois.justice.gc.ca/eng/regulations/C.R.C.%2C_c._870/.

C.08.005

(a) Subject to subsection (1.1) and notwithstanding Sections C.08.002 and C.08.003, a manufacturer of a new drug may sell it to a qualified investigator to be used solely for the purpose of clinical testing to obtain evidence with respect to the safety, dosage, and effectiveness of that new drug, when the following conditions are met:
(1) before the sale, the manufacturer has filed with the Minister, in compliance with Section C.08.005.1, a preclinical submission containing information and material respecting
(A) the brand name of the new drug or the identifying name or code proposed for the new drug,

(B) the chemical structure or other specific identification of the composition of the new drug,
(C) the source of the new drug,
(D) a detailed protocol of the clinical testing,
(E) the results of investigations made to support the clinical use of the new drug,
(F) the contraindications and precautions known in respect of the new drug and the suggested treatment of overdosage of the new drug,
(G) all ingredients of the new drug, stated quantitatively,
(H) the methods, equipment, plant and controls used in the manufacture, and processing and packaging of the new drug,
(I) the tests applied to control the potency, purity, and safety of the new drug, and
(J) the names and qualifications of all investigators to whom the drug is to be sold and the names of all institutions in which the clinical testing is to be carried out;

For the complete information about this rule please consult the following link: http://laws-lois.justice.gc.ca/eng/regulations/C.R.C.%2C_c._870/.

C.08.006

(a) For the purposes of this section, evidence or new information obtained by the Minister includes any information or material filed by any person pursuant to Division 5 or Sections C.08.002, C.08.002.01, C.08.002.1, C.08.003, C.08.005, or C.08.005.1.

(b) The Minister may, by notice to a manufacturer, suspend, for a definite or indefinite period, a notice of compliance issued to that manufacturer in respect of a new drug submission, an extraordinary use new drug submission, an abbreviated new drug submission, an abbreviated extraordinary use new drug submission, or a supplement to any of those submissions, if the Minister considers

(1) that the drug is not safe for the use represented in the submission or supplement, as shown by evidence obtained from

(A) clinical or other experience not reported in the submission or supplement or not available to the Minister at the time the notice of compliance was issued, or
(B) tests by new methods or tests by methods not reasonably applicable at the time the notice of compliance was issued;

(2) that, on the basis of new information obtained after the issuance of the notice of compliance, there is lack of substantial evidence that the drug will have the effect it is represented to have under the conditions of use prescribed, recommended, or proposed by the manufacturer;

(3) that the submission or supplement contained an untrue statement of material fact;

(4) that the manufacturer has failed to establish a system for maintaining required records or has repeatedly or deliberately failed to maintain such records;

(5) that, on the basis of new information obtained after the issuance of the notice of compliance, the methods, equipment, plant and controls used in the manufacturing, and processing and packaging of the drug are inadequate to assure and preserve the identity, strength, quality, or purity of the new drug;

(6) that, on the basis of new information obtained after the issuance of the notice of compliance, the labeling of the drug is false or misleading or incomplete in any manner and that this defect was not corrected by the manufacturer on receipt of a written notice from the Director specifying the respect in which the labeling is false or misleading or incomplete; or

(7) that, in the case of a new drug for extraordinary use, the manufacturer has not adhered to the plan referred to in subparagraph C.08.002.01(2) (b) (ix).

Annex 4

Resources for Readers

Begaud B. *Dictionary of Pharmacoepidemiology*. John Wiley & Sons Ltd; 2000.

CIOMS Working Group Pharmacovigilance. 2016. Available at: https://cioms.ch/pharmacovigilance/becoming-the-cioms-member/.

Cochrane Handbook for Systematic Reviews of Interventions. Available at: http://training.cochrane.org/handbook.

Committee for proprietary medicinal products (CPMP). *Points to Consider on Switching between Superiority and Non-inferiority*; 2000. Available at: http://www.ema.europa.eu/docs/en_GB/document_library/Scientific_guideline/2009/09/WC500003658.pdf.

EMA. *Points to Consider on Switching between Superiority and Non-inferiority*; 2000. Available at: www.ema.europa.eu/docs/en_GB/document/09/WC500003658.pdf.

The European Network of Centers for Pharmacoepidemiology and Pharmacovigilance (ENCePP). Guide on Methodological Standards in Pharmacoepidemiology (Revision 3). EMA/95,098/2010. Available at: http://www.encepp.eu/standards_and_guidances.

European Medicines Agency. *Guideline on the Use of Statistical Signal Detection Methods in the Eudravigilance Data Analysis System*; June 2008. http://www.ema.europa.eu/docs/en_GB/document_library/Regulatory_and_procedural_guideline/2009/11/WC500011434.pdf.

Food and Drug Act. Available at: http://laws-lois.justice.gc.ca/eng/acts/F-27.

Food and Drug Administration (FDA). *Guidance for Industry: Good Pharmacovigilance Practices and Pharmacoepidemiologic Assessment*; March 2005. http://www.fda.gov/downloads/RegulatoryInformation/Guidances/UCM126834.pdf.

Food and Drug Administration (FDA). *Guidance for Industry and FDA Staff: Best Practices for Conducting and Reporting Pharmacoepidemiologic Safety Studies Using Electronic Healthcare Data*; May 2013. Available at: http://www.fda.gov/downloads/Drugs/GuidanceComplianceRegulatoryInformation/Guidances/UCM243537.pdf.

Food and Drug Regulations. Available at: http://laws-lois.justice.gc.ca/eng/regulations/C.R.C.%2C_c._870/index.html.

Guidance Document. Pre-market Evaluation of Hepatotoxicity in Health Products. Available at: http://www.hc-sc.gc.ca/dhp-mps/prodpharma/applic-demande/guide-ld/hepatotox_guide_ld-eng.php.

Guidance Document. Conduct and Analysis of Comparative Bioavailability Studies. http://www.hc-sc.gc.ca/dhp-mps/prodpharma/applic-demande/guide-ld/bio/gd_cbs_ebc_ld-eng.php.

Guidance Document. Information and Submission Requirements for Biosimilar Biological Drugs. http://www.hc-sc.gc.ca/dhp-mps/brgtherap/applic-demande/guides/biosimilars-biosimilaires-eng.php.

Health Canada Risk Management Framework at the following link: http://www.hc-sc.gc.ca/ahc-asc/pubs/hpfb-dgpsa/risk-risques_tc-tm-eng.php.

Health Canada. *Inspection Strategy for Clinical Trials*; 2002. Available at: http://www.hc-sc.gc.ca/dhp-mps/compli-conform/clini-pract-prat/docs/insp_strat-eng.php.

Health Canada. *Good Manufacturing Practices (GMP) Guidelines - 2009 Edition, Version 2 (GUI-0001)*; 2009. Available at: http://www.hc-sc.gc.ca/dhp-mps/compli-conform/gmp-bpf/docs/gui-0001-eng.php.

Health Canada. *Post-notice of Compliance (NOC) Changes: Safety and Efficacy Document*; 2009. Available at: http://www.hc-sc.gc.ca/dhp-mps/prodpharma/applic-demande/guide-ld/postnoc_change_apresac/noc_pn_saf_ac_sa_inn-eng.php.

Health Canada. *Good Pharmacovigilance Practices (GVP) Guidelines (GUI-0102)*; 2011. Available at: http://www.hc-sc.gc.ca/dhp-mps/compli-conform/gmp-bpf/docs/gui-0102_gvp-eng.php.

Health Canada. *Good Pharmacovigilance Practices (GPP) Guidelines (GUI-0102)*; 2011. Available at: http://www.hc-sc.gc.ca/dhp-mps/compli-conform/gmp-bpf/docs/gui-0102_gvp-eng.php.

Health Canada. *Guidance for Industry: Management of Drug Submissions*; 2011. Available at: http://www.hc-sc.gc.ca/dhp-mps/prodpharma/applic-demande/guide-ld/mgmt-gest/mands_gespd-eng.php.

Health Canada. *Health Product Vigilance Framework*; 2012. Available at: http://www.hc-sc.gc.ca/dhp-mps/pubs/medeff/_fs-if/2012-hpvf-cvps/index-eng.php.

Health Canada. *Guidance Document for Clinical Trial Sponsors: Clinical Trial Applications*; 2013. Available at: http://www.hc-sc.gc.ca/dhp-mps/prodpharma/applic-demande/guide-ld/clini/ctdcta_ctddec-eng.php.

Health Canada. *Inspection Strategy for Good Pharmacovigilance Practices (GVP) for Drugs (POL-0041)*; 2013. Available at: http://www.hc-sc.gc.ca/dhp-mps/compli-conform/gmp-bpf/docs/pol-0041_gvp-eng.php.

Health Canada. *Regulatory Initiative: Regulations Amending the* Food and Drug Regulations—*orphan Drugs—forward Regulatory Plan 2016–2018*; 2016. Available at: http://www.hc-sc.gc.ca/ahc-asc/legislation/acts-reg-lois/frp-ppr/2016-2018/odrd-momr-eng.php.

Health Canada. *Products Monograph Guidance for Industry: Product Monograph*; 2017. Available at: http://www.hc-sc.gc.ca/dhp-mps/prodpharma/applic-demande/guide-ld/label_guide_ld-eng.php.

Health Canada: Good Pharmacovigilance Practices (GVP) Guidelines (GUI-0102). 2013. Available at: https://www.canada.ca/content/dam/hc-sc/migration/hc-sc/dhp-mps/alt_formats/pdf/compli-conform/gmp-bpf/docs/gui-0102_gvp-eng.pdf.

ICH guideline E2B (R3) on electronic transmission of individual case safety reports (ICSRs) - data elements and message specification - implementation guide. 2013. Available at: http://www.ema.europa.eu/docs/en_GB/document_library/Scientific_guideline/2009/09/WC500002767.pdf.

ICH Harmonised Tripartite Guideline. *Preclinical Safety Evaluation of Biotechnology-Derived Pharmaceuticals (S6 (R1))*; 2011. Disponible à: http://www.ich.org/fileadmin/Public_Web_Site/ICH_Products/Guidelines/Safety/S6_R1/Step4/S6_R1_Guideline.pdf.

ICH Harmonized Tripartite Guideline. *Clinical Safety Data Management: Definitions and Standards for Expedited Reporting E2A*; 1994. Disponible à http://www.ich.org/fileadmin/Public_Web_Site/ICH_Products/Guidelines/Efficacy/E2A/Step4/E2A_Guideline.pdf.

ICH Harmonized Tripartite Guideline. *Statistical Principal for Clinical Trials (E9)*; 1998. Disponible à: http://www.ich.org/fileadmin/Public_Web_Site/ICH_Products/Guidelines/Efficacy/E9/Step4/E9_Guideline.pdf.

ICH Harmonized Tripartite Guideline. *Good Manufacturing Practice Guide for Active Pharmaceutical Ingredients (Q7)*; 2000. Disponible à: http://www.ich.org/fileadmin/Public_Web_Site/ICH_Products/Guidelines/Quality/Q7/Step4/Q7_Guideline.pdf.

ICH Harmonized Tripartite Guideline. *Guidance on Non-clinical Safety Studies for the Conduct of Human Clinical Trials and Marketing Authorization for Pharmaceuticals (M3R2)*; 2009. Disponible à: http://www.ich.org/products/guidelines/multidisciplinary/article/multidisciplinary-guidelines.html.

ICH Harmonized Tripartite Guideline. *Guideline for Good Clinical Practice E6 (R1)*; 1996. Available at: http://www.ich.org/fileadmin/Public_Web_Site/ICH_Products/Guidelines/Efficacy/E6_R1/Step4/E6_R1__Guideline.pdf.

ICH Harmonized Tripartite Guideline. *Clinical Safety Data Management: Definitions and Standards for Expedited Reporting E2A*; 1994. Available à: http://www.ich.org/fileadmin/Public_Web_Site/ICH_Products/Guidelines/Efficacy/E2A/Step4/E2A_Guideline.pdf.

ICH Harmonized Tripartite Guideline. *Choice of Control Group and Related Issues in Clinical Trials (E10)*; 2000. Available at: www.ich.org//choice-of-control-group-and-related-issues-in-clinical-trials.pdf.

ICH Topic E 3: Structure and Content of Clinical Study Reports. 1996. Available at: http://www.ema.europa.eu/docs/en_GB/document_library/Scientific_guideline/2009/09/WC500002832.pdf.

International Society for Pharmacoepidemiology (ISPE). *Guidelines for Good Pharmacoepidemiology Practices (GPP)*. Pharmacoepidemiology and Drug Safety; 2008. Available at: http://www.pharmacoepi.org/pub/1c2a23af-2354-d714-516a-7175549e3a88.

Medical Devices Regulations. Available at: http://laws-lois.justice.gc.ca/eng/regulations/SOR-98-282/index.html.

OCDE. *OECD Principles on Good Laboratory Practice*; 1998. Available at: http://www.oecd-ilibrary.org/environment/oecd-principles-on-good-laboratory-practice_9789264078536-en.

QT/QTc Interval Prolongation. Guidance for Product Monograph Content. Available at: http://www.hc-sc.gc.ca/dhp-mps/prodpharma/applic-demande/guide-ld/qtqtc/qt_pm_mp-eng.php.

Rothman KJ, Greenland S, Lash TL. In: Rothman KJ, ed. *Modern Epidemiology*. 3rd ed. Philadelphia, PA: Lippincott, Williams & Wilkins; 2008.

Samet JM, Wipfli H, Platz EA, Bavspar N. *A Dictionary of Epidemiology*. Fifth Edition: Edited by Miquel Porta. *Am J Epidemiol*. 2009, 170:1449.

Strom B, Kimmel S, Hennessy S, eds. *Textbook of Pharmacoepidemiology*. 2nd ed. Sussex: John Wiley & Sons; 2013.

World Health Organization. Available at: http://www.who.int/topics/epidemiology/en/.

Index

'*Note*: Page numbers followed by "f" indicate figures and "t" indicate tables.'

FSC
www.fsc.org
MIX
Papier | Fördert
gute Waldnutzung
FSC® C083411

Kolibri 360 GmbH
Ferdinand-Jühlke-Straße 7
99095 Erfurt, Deutschland
produktsicherheit@kolibri360.de